T0226606

Rheumatology—A Survival Guide for the Primary Care Physician

Guest Editor

R. ALLEN PERKINS, MD, MPH

PRIMARY CARE: CLINICS IN OFFICE PRACTICE

www.primarycare.theclinics.com

Consulting Editor
JOEL J. HEIDELBAUGH, MD

December 2010 • Volume 37 • Number 4

SAUNDERS an imprint of ELSEVIER, Inc.

W.B. SAUNDERS COMPANY
A Division of Elsevier Inc.

1600 John F. Kennedy Boulevard, Suite 1800 • Philadelphia, PA 19103-2899

http://www.theclinics.com

PRIMARY CARE: CLINICS IN OFFICE PRACTICE Volume 37, Number 4
December 2010 ISSN 0095-4543, ISBN-13: 978-1-4377-2490-5

Editor: Barbara Cohen-Kligerman
Developmental Editor: Donald Mumford

Primary Care: Clinics in Office Practice (ISSN: 0095–4543) is published quarterly by Elsevier Inc., 360 Park Avenue South, New York, NY 10010-1710. Months of issue are March, June, September, and December. Periodicals postage paid at New York, NY and additional mailing offices. Subscription prices are $203.00 per year (US individuals), $336.00 (US institutions), $101.00 (US students), $248.00 (Canadian individuals), $395.00 (Canadian institutions), $159.00 (Canadian students), $309.00 (international individuals), $395.00 (international institutions), and $159.00 (international students). Foreign air speed delivery is included in all *Clinics* subscription prices. All prices are subject to change without notice. POSTMASTER: Send address changes to *Primary Care: Clinics in Office Practice*, Elsevier Periodicals Customer Service, 11830 Westline Industrial Drive, St. Louis, MO 63146. Customer Service Health Sciences Division, Subscription Customer Service, 3251 Riverport Lane, Maryland Heights, MO 63043. **Customer Service: 1-800-654-2452 (U.S. and Canada); 314-447-8871 (outside U.S. and Canada). Fax: 314-447-8029. E-mail: journalscustomerservice-usa@elsevier.com (for print support); journalsonlinesupport-usa@elsevier.com (for online support).**

Reprints. For copies of 100 or more, of articles in this publication, please contact the Commercial Reprints Department, Elsevier Inc., 360 Park Avenue South, New York, NY 10010-1710. Tel. (212) 633-3812; Fax: (212) 482-1935; E-mail: reprints@elsevier.com.

Primary Care: Clinics in Office Practice is covered in *MEDLINE/PubMed (Index Medicus) and EMBASE/ Excerpta Medica, Current Contents/Clinical Medicine, and ISI/BIOMED.*

Printed and bound by CPI Group (UK) Ltd, Croydon, CR0 4YY

Transferred to Digital Print 2011

Contributors

CONSULTING EDITOR

JOEL J. HEIDELBAUGH, MD
Clinical Assistant Professor and Clerkship Director, Department of Family Medicine; Clinical Assistant Professor, Department of Urology, University of Michigan Medical School, Ann Arbor, Michigan

GUEST EDITOR

R. ALLEN PERKINS, MD, MPH
Professor and Chair, Department of Family Medicine, University of South Alabama, Mobile, Alabama

AUTHORS

R. BRIAN BETTENCOURT, MD
Family Medicine Residency Program, University of South Alabama, Mobile, Alabama

SHELLEY BHATTACHARYA, DO, MPH
Department of Family Medicine, Division of Geriatric Medicine & Palliative Care, University of Kansas School of Medicine, Kansas City, Kansas

JAMES T. BIRCH JR, MD, MSPH
Department of Family Medicine, Division of Geriatric Medicine & Palliative Care, University of Kansas School of Medicine, Kansas City, Kansas

R. LAMAR DUFFY, MD
Assistant Professor of Medicine, Department of Family Medicine, University of South Alabama, Mobile, Alabama

ZEWDU HAILE, MD
Faculty, Hinsdale Family Medicine Residency, Hinsdale, Illinois

NATASHA HARDER, MD
Assistant Residency Director, Tuscaloosa Family Medicine Residency; Assistant Professor, Department of Family Medicine, University of Alabama School of Medicine, Tuscaloosa, Alabama

SANJEEB KHATUA, MD
Chief Resident, Hinsdale Family Medicine Residency, Hinsdale, Illinois

CHARLES KODNER, MD
Associate Professor, Department of Family and Geriatric Medicine, University of Louisville School of Medicine, Louisville, Kentucky

MICHAEL M. LINDER, MD
Associate Professor of Family Medicine, Family Medicine Residency Program, University of South Alabama, Mobile, Alabama

MEREDITH L. MAXWELL, MD, MHA
Department of Family Medicine, University of South Alabama, Mobile, Alabama

JOSEPH P. MICHALSKI, MD
Professor, Department of Internal Medicine, University of South Alabama, Mobile, Alabama

EHAB A. MOLOKHIA, MD
Associate Professor, Department of Family Medicine, University of South Alabama; Medical Director, USA Family Practice Clinic, Mobile, Alabama

CAROL P. MOTLEY, MD
Associate Professor, Department of Family Medicine, University of South Alabama, Mobile, Alabama

DAVID M. QUILLEN, MD
Associate Professor, Department of Community Health and Family Medicine, University of Florida, Gainesville, Florida

JOHN B. WAITS, MD
Program Director, Tuscaloosa Family Medicine Residency Program; Associate Professor, Department of Family Medicine / Obstetrics and Gynecology, College of Community Health Sciences, University of Alabama School of Medicine, Tuscaloosa, Alabama

Contents

The rational use of laboratory testing to investigate early, undifferentiated joint pain depends heavily on a detailed history and careful physical examination. Nevertheless, several diagnostic tests have some discriminatory function in the initial evaluation of soft tissues and joint complaints, given the correct clinical context. Arthrocentesis frequently gives the best results when compared with other tests in the differential diagnosis of monoarticular and polyarticular joint pain. There is also a role for radiographs, and less frequently, magnetic resonance imaging. Although overuse of an arthritis panel is not recommended, for an appropriately chosen patient, complete blood cell count, serum uric acid, C-reactive protein (or erythrocyte sedimentation rate), rheumatoid factor, antiecyclic citrullinated peptide, and antinuclear antibody titers form a reasonable screening panel when rheumatic disease is suspected based on the clinical condition. Other tests might include a purified protein derivative, anti-Borrelia titers, and antibodies for antistreptolysin O. However, many rheumatic conditions can be diagnosed or at least suspected on clinical grounds alone, and a careful history and physical examination are absolutely essential for the appropriate use of any laboratory testing.

Athrocentesis and therapeutic joint injection is a safe and useful primary care procedure. Fluid collection and analysis from effused joints is important to establish a cause and therefore inform appropriate management. Therapeutic joint injection can give patients significant, rapid, localized pain relief.

Gout is a common disease and the prevalence is increasing. Chronic hyperuricemia (uric acid serum levels >6.8 mg/dL) is a key feature. Treating to a target uric acid level of 6.0 mg/dL is recommended. In addition to cochicine, probenecid, and allopurinol, feboxostat is a new option for urate-lowering therapy.

> About 15% of patients presenting in a primary care clinic have joint pain as their primary complaint (level B). Disseminated gonorrhea is the most common cause of infectious arthritis in sexually active, previously healthy patients (level B). Prompt arthrocentesis, microscopic examination, and the culture of any purulent material plus appropriate antibiotic therapy are the mainstay of treatment in infectious arthritis (level C). Detailed history, including family history and comprehensive examination, is more useful in accurate diagnosis than expensive laboratory and radiological investigations for noninfectious arthritis (level C). Regarding inflammatory noninfectious arthritis with the potential to cause destructive joint damage, early referral to a subspecialist, when indicated, increases the likelihood of optimal outcome (level C). Nonsteroidal antiinflammatory drugs are the first line of therapeutic agents to reduce pain and swelling in the management of most noninfectious inflammatory arthritis seen in the primary care office (level C).

> Low back pain is a common condition, responsible for significant morbidity and major occupational and economic impact on society. While most cases of low back pain spontaneously resolve, the clinician must be alert to clinical indicators or "red flags" that suggest the presence of systemic illness or imminent neurologic compromise. In the absence of such findings, diagnostic imaging generally does not contribute to management, and may be safely delayed for a trial of conservative therapy. Continued activity is associated with a favorable outcome. Nonsteroidal anti-inflammatories, acetaminophen, muscle relaxants, and tricyclic antidepressants can provide meaningful pain relief, while several nonpharmacologic measures may also contribute to symptomatic and functional improvement.

> In caring for the patient with fibromyalgia, the primary care provider benefits from an understanding of fibromyalgia as a distinct entity. Evidence-based diagnostic criteria for fibromyalgia can be used in all individuals who present with multiple site pain, fatigue, and poor sleep. Planning therapy for individuals with fibromyalgia often involves using both pharmacologic and nonpharmacologic treatment in the primary care setting.

> Temporal arteritis, also known as giant cell arteritis, is the most common vasculitis in adults. Classic symptoms include polymyalgia rheumatica, new-onset headache, jaw claudication, and visual symptoms such as

diplopia and amaurosis fugax. Elevated erythrocyte sedimentation rate is a common laboratory finding in temporal arteritis, and abnormalities on temporal artery biopsy are the gold standard for diagnosis. Rapid treatment with steroids can prevent permanent vision loss, which is the worst ischemic complication of the disease. It is important for primary care physicians to be able to recognize the signs and symptoms of this disease and begin treatment rapidly.

Systemic lupus erythematosus is an autoimmune inflammatory disorder that frequently affects women of childbearing age. A diagnosis is made by confirming the presence of at least 4 of 11 criteria proposed by the American College of Rheumatology. Almost all patients should take hydroxychloroquine and most require corticosteroids, with immunosuppressive drugs frequently given as well. With better management, patients with lupus live longer but are at increased risk of disease and treatment-related complications, including infection, cardiovascular disease, and osteoporosis. These problems should be monitored and treated in the primary care setting.

Rheumatoid arthritis is an inflammatory disease of the joints causing pain and stiffness, pathologically characterized by chronic synovitis. Without proper treatment, it progresses to cause joint deformity that results in significant loss of function. Extra-articular disease can also occur, which exacerbates morbidity and mortality associated with the disease. Patients from all age groups can acquire the disease, hence the additional categories of juvenile onset and elderly onset rheumatoid arthritis. Disease-modifying antirheumatic drugs are the mainstay of therapy, and should be initiated as early as possible in the course of the disease in consultation with a rheumatologist.

Many serious adverse events and complications may occur in patients with rheumatologic diseases. Such adverse events and complications may be a direct complication of the disease process or a result of the medications used for the therapy. Primary care physicians are frequently involved in the management of these patients. It is therefore necessary for them to be aware of the currently available recommendations to monitor for adverse events. It is through the understanding of these recommendations and their successful implementation in practice that primary care physicians will contribute to improved patient outcomes.

FORTHCOMING ISSUES

March 2011
Substance Abuse in Office-Based Practice
Robert Mallin, MD,
Guest Editor

June 2011
Palliative Care
Serife Eti Karakas, MD,
Guest Editor

September 2011
Gastrointestinal Disease
James Winger, MD, and
Aaron Michelfelder, MD, FAAFP,
Guest Editors

RECENT ISSUES

September 2010
Primary Care Urology
Karl T. Rew, MD, and
Masahito Jimbo, MD, PhD, MPH, MD,
Guest Editors

June 2010
Integrative Medicine in Primary Care, Part II:
Disease States and Body Systems
Roger Zoorob, MD, MPH, FAAFP,
and Vincent Morelli, MD,
Guest Editors

March 2010
Integrative Medicine, Part I: Incorporating
Complementary/Alternative Modalities
J. Adam Rindfleisch, MD, MPhil,
Guest Editor

ISSUES OF RELATED INTEREST

Pediatric Clinics of North America, June 2010 (Vol. 57, Issue 3)
Adolescents and Sports
Dilip R. Patel, MD, and Donald E. Greydanus, MD, FSAM, FIAP (H), *Guest Editors*
Available at: http://www.pediatric.theclinics.com/

Clinics in Geriatric Medicine, May 2010 (Vol. 26, Issue 2)
The Aging Male
John E. Morley, MB, BCh, *Guest Editor*
Available at: http://www.geriatric.theclinics.com/

VISIT THE CLINICS ONLINE!

Access your subscription at:
www.theclinics.com

Foreword

Providing a Road Map to Survive Rheumatologic Disease

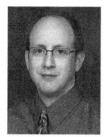

Joel J. Heidelbaugh, MD
Consulting Editor

Over a year ago when I asked Dr Allen Perkins to embark upon creating a volume of *Primary Care: Clinics in Office Practice* to serve as a rheumatology primer for primary care clinicians, I don't think that either one of us initially appreciated the scope or magnitude of what was really required for such a project to be effective. I asked Dr Perkins to consider compiling a series of evidence-based articles that would help us approach patients with ambiguous complaints such as fatigue, myalgias, arthralgias, weakness, and other such symptoms that we hear about on a daily basis but are often challenged to approach in a time- and cost-effective fashion. When I heard his ideas for a "survival guide," my imagination quickly referenced the popular television show *Survivor*, somehow drawing a parallel between both the clinician and the patient trying to understand and cope with the inherent challenges of managing and living with these confusing disorders.

We know that self-reported quality of life among people with rheumatologic diseases is significantly lower than that of nonafflicted populations, as 40% of patients are more likely to report fair or poor general health; 30% are more likely to need help with personal care, and these individuals are twice as likely to have a health-related activity limitation affecting every domain of human activity, including work, leisure, and social relations.[1] However, many of today's primary care clinicians report that they are ill-equipped to diagnose and manage rheumatologic conditions in an effective fashion. This trend has led to the development of the theory that such patients could be cared for exclusively by rheumatologists.[2]

Prim Care Clin Office Pract 37 (2010) ix–xi
doi:10.1016/j.pop.2010.07.012   **primarycare.theclinics.com**

In trying to make sense of these complex symptoms, the following questions come to my mind when thinking about our daily practices with respect to rheumatologic diseases:

- Have you ever felt that you incompletely evaluated a patient who presented with one or more of the aforementioned symptoms, with regard to both laboratory tests and initial treatment?
- Have you ever ordered a battery of tests searching for a rheumatologic disorder, only to find that you couldn't adequately interpret them?
- Perhaps not infrequently, but have you ever referred a patient in whom you thought you had performed a complete initial serologic workup, only to find that the rheumatologist ordered tests that you've never thought of or heard of?
- Worse yet, have you ever referred a patient to a rheumatologist after completing a seemingly thorough negative workup only to have the specialist offer a diagnosis of a "seronegative" condition and not much hope for treatment?

Over the last few years, I've diagnosed more cases of fibromyalgia, lupus, rheumatoid arthritis, and Sjogren's syndrome than in the early years of my practice, and in beating statistics of prevalence and incidence, I recently diagnosed ankylosing spondylitis in 3 brothers of Palestinian heritage. As fibromyalgia is estimated to occur now in 2% of the US population, it often makes me feel that I must be underdiagnosing it! Nonetheless, despite current evidence-based recommendations to treat conditions such as fibromyalgia, many clinicians find themselves relying upon narcotic pain medications since other options may fail to provide and restore an acceptable level of functionality for our patients.

Another great challenge in rheumatology is learning about the pharmacologic options to treat these disorders. It seems as if our lay press and television commercials are inundating us with advertisements for novel therapies for rheumatoid arthritis, lupus, and other rheumatologic conditions. In 2009, retail costs for etanercept (Enbrel) and adalimumab (Humira) alone totaled over $2 billion.[3] While the promise of medications to treat symptoms of rheumatologic diseases to improve quality of life seems quite engaging, the potential side effects seem harrowing. Perhaps even more frightening is the prospect of primary care clinicians not having familiarity with such agents, yet being obligated to manage complex medical comorbidities and drug–drug interactions.

Dr Perkins and his authors deserve a world of recognition and gratitude for undertaking the gargantuan task of creating this unique volume of articles, a true "road map" to help both clinicians and patients survive the ambiguities and challenges of diagnosing, treating, and living with rheumatologic disease. What cannot be understated here is the increasing need for primary care clinicians to learn the complexities of evaluating and managing rheumatologic diseases, the pharmacokinetics and adverse effects of current and new biologic agents to treat these disorders, and the necessity of a strong and communicative relationship between the rheumatologist and the primary care clinician within the medical home model to promote better outcomes for our patients.

Joel J. Heidelbaugh, MD
Departments of Family Medicine and Urology
University of Michigan Medical School
Ann Arbor, MI 48109, USA

Ypsilanti Health Center
200 Arnet Street, Suite 200
Ypsilanti, MI 48198, USA

E-mail address:
jheidel@umich.edu

REFERENCES

1. Dominick KL, Ahern FM, Gold CH, et al. Health-related quality of life among older adults with arthritis. Health Qual Life Outcomes 2004;2(1):5.
2. Kaufman RL. The rheumatologist as principal care physician. Available at: http://www.lupusmd.org/docs/living-rheumatologist.html. Accessed July 18, 2010.
3. Drug Topics, Pharmacy Facts and Figures. Available at: http://drugtopics.modernmedicine.com/drugtopics/data/articlestandard//drugtopics/252010/674961/article.pdf. Accessed July 18, 2010.

Preface

Primary Care, Rheumatology, and the Medical Neighborhood

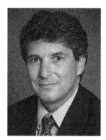

R. Allen Perkins, MD, MPH
Guest Editor

A practicing primary care physician will see a patient with a complaint associated with a rheumatologic condition on a daily basis. Eighteen percent of all physicians' visits are made because of such symptoms.[1] Musculoskeletal complaints are second only to hypertension as a reason for a physician's office visit in the United States. As the baby boomers pass retirement age, the number of these visits will only increase. Although many of these patients will have a chronic condition such as osteoarthritis that requires minimal attention in the course of a routine visit, rheumatologic complaints tend to cause physician anxiety (both warranted and unwarranted). The purpose of this guide is to help refocus some of this anxious energy into action.

The patient with an undifferentiated musculoskeletal complaint often presents as a diagnostic dilemma. Although clearly uncomfortable, the patient may have little or no objective findings and yet may eventually develop severe disease.[2] Development of an assessment strategy that includes familiarity with and referral for "red flags," rational use of diagnostic tests, and use of conservative management and watchful waiting will improve both patient and physician satisfaction. An enhanced relationship with the "partialists"[3] may result as a consequence of this as well.

Patients with a diagnosed rheumatic condition present another set of problems. They are often on a myriad of disease-modifying agents, and although they may have a very simple complaint, it can rapidly escalate into something more serious. In addition, patients may believe they are receiving good primary care when in fact none of their physicians are providing preventive services. Rheumatologists do not consider themselves to be primary care physicians and desire an improved working

Financial support: None.

Prim Care Clin Office Pract 37 (2010) xiii–xiv
doi:10.1016/j.pop.2010.07.011
0095-4543/10/$ – see front matter

relationship with the primary care team.[4] Achieving this has been a challenge in the current health care environment.

The Patient Centered Medical Home model offers a potential solution in the concept of the Medical Neighborhood.[5] Such a model would facilitate coordination of care and improve consultations and comanagement to create "seamless transitions" for patients. We can strive for this model; however, currently we need to learn as much as we can about our patients' illnesses and work to improve 2-way communications since patients with rheumatologic illnesses will continue to walk into the primary care practice with a complaint of "I'm sick."

With this issue, we present information relevant to caring for both types of patients. We present information on the diagnosis and management of patients with undifferentiated complaints. We also present evidence-based information on patients with rheumatologic illnesses that are individually rare but in aggregate are relatively common. While the management of these patients requires close contact with a rheumatologist, many of these patients seek out primary care for common complaints. Additionally, distance often requires collaboration between the rheumatologist and the primary care physician. We hope that this information allows the primary care physician to offer better care as well as to understand when to put a call to his or her neighbor.

As the guest editor, I want to express my thanks to these authors. All of them are too busy to have said yes but did so anyway and despite other obligations managed to give me some outstanding manuscripts. They are caring for these patients and felt it was important to share their knowledge with you. I also want to thank Barbara Cohen-Kligerman, the managing editor, and the rest of the staff who put up with a bunch of busy physicians and their excuses.

R. Allen Perkins, MD, MPH
Department of Family Medicine
University of South Alabama
1504 Springhill Avenue, Suite 3414
Mobile, AL 36604, USA

E-mail address:
perkins@usouthal.edu

REFERENCES

1. Cherry DK, Woodwell DA, Rechtsteiner EA. National Ambulatory Medical Care Survey: 2005 Summary. Advance data from vital and health statistics: no. 387. Hyattsville (MD): National Center for Health Statistics; 2007.
2. Adib N. Association between duration of symptoms and severity of disease at first presentation to paediatric rheumatology: results from the Childhood Arthritis Prospective Study. Rheumatology (Oxford) 2008;47(7):991–5.
3. Duane M. Breaking from tradition: refocusing the locus of family medicine training—reaction to the paper by Perry A. Pugno, MD, MPH. J Am Board Fam Med 2010;23:S30–1.
4. Wallace DJ. Improving the prognosis of SLE without prescribing lupus drugs and the primary care paradox. Lupus 2008;17(2):91–2.
5. Starfield B. Primary care, specialist care, and chronic care: can they interlock? Chest 2010;137:8–10.

Rational Use of Laboratory Testing in the Initial Evaluation of Soft Tissue and Joint Complaints

John B. Waits, MD*

KEYWORDS

- Rheumatology • Early undifferentiated joint pain • Arthritis
- Laboratory workup • Monoarticular • Polyarticular
- Arthrocentesis • Anti–cyclic citrullinated peptide

Joint pain is a ubiquitous chief complaint in clinical primary care, encompassing initial workup and primary management of the various arthritides. Therapeutic intervention performed by primary care includes pharmaceutical and procedural approaches. Occasionally, medical and surgical referral and comanagement are warranted. An efficient and accurate workup of early, undifferentiated joint pain for discrimination in the wide differential diagnosis of arthritis is essential. This is made possible by the continued development of and clinical experience with disease-modifying agents for rheumatoid arthritis (RA) and other rheumatologic diseases in which early diagnosis and intervention is proving to be beneficial.

Unfortunately, rarely does "laboratory studies provide the diagnosis in joint pain."[1] The classic example of this is rheumatoid factor (RF), which is negative in as many as 25% to 30% of total RA cases—and is possibly negative in up to 50% of early cases of RA.[1–3] Conversely, the RF can be falsely positive in the absence of RA, particularly in certain disease states, such as bacterial endocarditis, other chronic indolent infections, interstitial pulmonary fibrosis, and primary biliary cirrhosis,[4] and even as a part of normal aging.

Given these limitations in the face of an extensive differential diagnosis for acute undifferentiated joint pain, the importance of pretest probability—clinical judgment and likelihood based on history and physical examination—becomes clear. Simply

Tuscaloosa Family Medicine Residency Program, Department of Family Medicine/Obstetrics and Gynecology, College of Community Health Sciences, University of Alabama School of Medicine, 850 5th Avenue East, Box 870377, Tuscaloosa, AL 35487-0377, USA
* Corresponding author.
E-mail address: jwaits@cchs.ua.edu

Prim Care Clin Office Pract 37 (2010) 673–689
doi:10.1016/j.pop.2010.07.010
0095-4543/10/$ – see front matter © 2010 Published by Elsevier Inc.

Key Points	Evidence Rating
Laboratory testing should not be undertaken in the absence of a careful history and physical examination, establishing the pretest probability of disease	B
Arthrocentesis and subsequent examination of the synovial fluid have high accuracy and discriminatory power between various differential diagnoses in both monoarticular and polyarticular presentations in appropriately chosen patients	B
Osteoarthritis can be diagnosed on clinical grounds alone	B
Radiographs should be considered for acute joint pain with a history of injury or trauma and chronic joint pain	C
A reasonable arthritis panel ordered after a careful history, physical examination, appropriate radiography, and arthrocentesis might include	
Complete blood cell count	
Uric acid	
C-Reactive protein (CRP) or erythrocyte sedimentation rate (ESR)	
Rheumatoid factor (RF)	
Anti–cyclic citrullinated peptide (anti-CCP)	
Antinuclear antibodies (ANA) with reflex	
PPD, anti-Borrelia (Lyme) titers, and antistreptolysin O may be useful in the appropriate settings	C
Thirty percent of patients with rheumatoid arthritis (RA) are seronegative for RF	A
Ordering anti-CCP along with the RF increases the sensitivity of detecting early RA	A
Many people with active RA have relatively normal values of ESR or CRP and many with quiescent RA have abnormal values	A
Uric acid can be normal even in an acute gout attack	B
Serum uric acid should be measured 2 weeks after a presumed gout attack to test for elevation	B
Low-level ANA titers greater than or equal to a ratio of 1:40 are seen in up to 20% to 30% of healthy individuals and this increases with age	A
ANA titers with specific antibodies should be measured only when ANA-related diseases are highly suspected on clinical grounds	B

stated, it is rarely possible to rule in or rule out these conditions without careful clinical judgment.

HISTORY

The cornerstone of careful clinical judgment is an efficient and detailed history. The following key points are worth reviewing for enhancing the history of present illness in the setting of a musculoskeletal chief complaint: pain, stiffness, limitation of motion, swelling, weakness, and fatigue (**Table 1**).[5]

No scored combination of clinical features (similar to the Well criteria for deep vein thrombosis, for instance) has yet been validated to give firm, evidence-based guidance toward the use of laboratory tests in discerning the rheumatologic cause of musculoskeletal complaints. However, keeping the historical components of the

Table 1
Key points of the history

History	Details
Pain	Description, onset, location, patterns of progression, severity, and exacerbating and alleviating factors
Stiffness	Time of day and clinical setting (eg, early morning vs after activity), and duration
Limitation of Motion	Location, duration, rapidity of onset, passive vs active, interval history, and responsiveness to previous interventions
Swelling	Location, duration, and clinical course
Weakness	Onset, duration, and distribution
Fatigue	Historical pattern and context

From Firestein GS, Budd RC, Harris ED Jr, et al. Kelley's textbook of rheumatology. 8th edition. Philadelphia: W.B. Saunders; 2008; with permission.

diagnostic criteria of the most common rheumatologic complaints at the forefront of one's mind not only guides and expedites a rational history and examination but also guides the rational ordering of laboratory testing.

PHYSICAL EXAMINATION

As in many other clinical conditions, history is critical in establishing the pretest likelihood of rheumatologic disease. Physical examination is seldom as important and useful as in the musculoskeletal system, particularly in establishing the pretest probability of an eventual diagnosis of early, undifferentiated arthritis. The following specific components of the physical examination are recapitulated here: swelling, tenderness, limitation of motion, crepitation, deformity, and instability (**Table 2**).[5]

DIAGNOSTIC INVESTIGATIONS

Every diagnostic test has a unique series of characteristics that indicate its accuracy in a given context.[6–8]

Table 2
Key points of physical examination

Components of Physical Examination	Details
Swelling	Articular vs synovial vs periarticular; symmetry
Tenderness	Articular vs periarticular; are there other myofacial tender points?
Limitation of Motion	Range of motion; passive vs active
Crepitation	Character of crepitation; which joints?
Deformity	Character of deformity; which joints?
Instability	Which joints?

From Firestein GS, Budd RC, Harris ED Jr, et al. Kelley's textbook of rheumatology. 8th edition. Philadelphia: W.B. Saunders; 2008; with permission.

Sensitivity and specificity are 2 of the most basic characteristics of a diagnostic test. Both are independent of the prevalence of the disease in question.

Sensitivity describes the ability of a diagnostic test to identify true disease without missing anyone by leaving the disease undiagnosed. Thus, a high sensitivity test has few false negatives and is effective at ruling conditions "out" (SnOut).

Specificity describes the ability of a diagnostic test to be correctly negative in the absence of disease without mislabeling anyone. Thus, a high specificity test has few false positives and is effective in ruling conditions "in" (SpIn).

Both report features of a given diagnostic test that are independent of the actual prevalence of the disease. However, because clinicians typically practice with the explicit or implicit knowledge of disease prevalence, the positive and negative predictive values (PPV and NPV, respectively) of tests are often more useful than raw sensitivity and specificity.

NPV puts sensitivity into the context of known disease prevalence by reporting the "probability that an individual is not affected with the condition when a negative test result is observed" National Cancer Institute (NCI).

$$NPV = (True\ negative)/(True\ and\ false\ negatives)$$

PPV puts specificity into the context of known disease prevalence by reporting the "probability that an individual is affected with the condition when a positive test result is observed" [NCI].

$$PPV = (True\ positive)/(True\ and\ false\ positives)$$

Taking a different slant, likelihood ratios express the relative odds that a positive test represents a correct clinical diagnosis or true positive (LR+) and that a negative test represents a true negative (LR−). Likelihood ratios greater than 5 and less than 0.2 are typically the most clinically relevant.

$$LR+ = (Test\ sensitivity)/(1 - Test\ specificity)LR- = (1 - Test\ sensitivity)/(Test\ specificity)$$

To illustrate these concepts, suppose that over the past few months 200 patients were seen and ordered a standing 2-view knee radiograph. For the sake of discussion, the radiograph has a sensitivity of 80% and a specificity of 90% for osteoarthritis (OA) and the prevalence of OA is 15 in 100 (15%) in the population (**Table 3**).

Among the 30 patients who prove to eventually have true OA, the initial standing knee radiograph was positive in only 24, leaving 6 with a false-negative result. This, [24/(6+24)], illustrates an 80% sensitivity.

Table 3
Demonstration of how a moderately sensitive and specific test performs in the context of a disease with a high prevalence, such as OA (numbers simplified for demonstration purposes)

	OA Present	OA Absent	Total
Radiograph Positive	24	17	41
Radiograph Negative	6	153	159
Total	30	170	200

Similarly, among the 170 patients who later prove not to have true OA, the initial radiograph was negative in most (152), leaving 17 with a confusing false-positive result. This, [153/(17+153)], illustrates a 90% specificity (see **Table 3**).

Hence, the prevalence of OA in this population is 15% (30/200). Remembering that if the true prevalence of a disease is not known, the following equations cannot be used with certainty; the NPV of this radiograph for ruling out OA is 96% [153/(6+153)], and the PPV for diagnosing OA is about 59% [24/(24+17)].

Consider a hypothetical test for Sjögren syndrome with the same sensitivity and specificity (0.8 and 0.9, respectively) and a much lower (hypothetical) prevalence of 1 in 100 (**Table 4**).

In this circumstance (same test characteristics, lower prevalence), the NPV and PPV would be as follows:

NPV = 99.78% [900/(2 + 900)]PPV = 7.41% [8/(8 + 100)]

Thus, for rare diseases, the discriminatory power of a diagnostic test with reasonable sensitivity and specificity for ruling out a rare disease (ie, NPV) is robust. However, when diseases are rare, ruling in a test (ie, PPV) based on a single positive test is simply not possible. This theme has broad implications for most of the tests and conditions being discussed.

An online version of these tables and calculations is available.[9]

ARTHROCENTESIS

The most valuable laboratory test in sorting out early, undifferentiated arthritis, whether monoarticular or polyarticular in presentation, is an examination of the synovial fluid by arthrocentesis in the appropriately chosen patient. Every individual with a monoarticular effusion deserves at least 1 diagnostic arthrocentesis.[10,11]

Details on the procedural skill of arthrocentesis are available in several references.[10–13] Three considerations are germane in proceeding with arthrocentesis: indications, procedural skill, and order and interpret the synovial fluid analysis.

For further discussion on arthrocentesis, see the related article in this issue.

RADIOGRAPHS

Radiographic modalities should not be overlooked as a source of diagnostic information. Radiographs help observe and assess possible chronic changes from OA, calcium pyrophosphate dihydrate disease, RA, and gout.

In addition, many circumstances warrant the use of radiographs when there is a traumatic mechanism or injury or an acute onset of joint pain, particularly looking for acute fracture or avulsion. However, much evidence has been accumulated over the last 2

Table 4
Demonstration of how a moderately sensitive and specific test performs in the context of a disease with a low prevalence, such as Sjögren syndrome (numbers simplified for demonstration purposes)

	Sjögren Present	Sjögren Absent	Total
Test Positive	8	100	108
Test Negative	2	900	902
Total	10	1000	1010

decades regarding appropriate and potentially inappropriate use of radiographs, even in the face of acute trauma. In some of the most classic and seminal studies of multi-sign, multisymptom decision rules, the Ottawa Knee and Ankle Rules guide the clinician into when to order radiographs after acute knee and acute ankle injuries based on a simple list of clinically relevant historical symptoms and physical examination signs.[14–17]

Multiple guidelines from the American College of Radiology (ACR Appropriateness Criteria) exist regarding the imaging of joints in the face of chronic pain. They can be found at www.guideline.gov and include nontraumatic knee pain and chronic hip, elbow, ankle, foot, wrist, and neck pain.[18–24] All these recommend high correlation with the clinical situation (a recurring theme) and obtain plain radiographs as the initial image. Magnetic resonance imaging is warranted when the history and physical examination suggest occult fracture, tumor, ligamentous and meniscal injury, neurologic involvement, other internal derangements, or atypical osteomyelitis.

The usefulness of plain radiographs in diagnosing OA at the hip and knee has been estimated.[25] The sensitivity and specificity at the hip are 89% and 90% and at the knee, 83% and 93%, respectively. Given the high prevalence of OA in the general population, this provides a robust NPV of plain radiographs (>95%) but a limited PPV (<60%).

COMPLETE BLOOD CELL COUNT

One of the most common laboratory tests that is a part of any investigatory panel is the complete blood cell count (CBC). No definitive data exist regarding the overall usefulness of the CBC in ruling in or ruling out rheumatic disease, and most clinicians are familiar with the limitations of the white blood cell count (WBC) in the CBC in ruling in or ruling out any particular type of infection. Nevertheless, a few comments are worth mentioning.

The jWBC (joint white blood cell count) from an arthrocentesis is much more discriminatory than the serum WBC alone. Taken in isolation, the WBC is poor at ruling in or ruling out septic arthritis. The positive likelihood ratio (LR+) is 1.7 [95% confidence interval (CI), 1.2–2.3] and the negative likelihood ratio (LR−) is 0.46 (95% CI, 0.19–1.1).[26] Thus, the serum WBC alone is fairly unhelpful in ruling in or ruling out septic arthritis.

On the other hand, obtaining a CBC "may reveal anemia of chronic disease, or sometimes leukemia, that can be another cause of acute or chronic joint pain."[1] Therefore, the traditional course of including the CBC in the arthritis panel is probably worthwhile.

SERUM AND URINE URIC ACID

After OA, gout competes with RA as the most common rheumatic condition in primary care practice.[27,28] Therefore, understanding the role of serum uric acid and urine uric acid is important.

Like many tests that have been discussed, serum uric acid alone has poor discriminatory value. Many patients with an acute gout attack have a normal uric acid level. Conversely, many patients with no symptoms have an elevated uric acid level. Serum uric acid level has a PPV of only 22% if a cutoff of 9 mg/dL is used and less for a lower cutoff value, rendering it useless for predicting who will develop symptoms.[29]

ACUTE-PHASE REACTANTS
Erythrocyte Sedimentation Rate (SED Rate) and C-Reactive Protein

Erythrocyte sedimentation rate (ESR) and C-reactive protein (CRP) level are commonly elevated in inflammatory conditions, such as RA, septic joint,[1] osteomyelitis, polymyalgia rheumatica (PMR), and temporal arteritis, although the pathognomonic nature of the tests in the PMR, and temporal arteritis conditions has been called into question recently. In technical terms, ESR is the distance that erythrocytes (RBCs) fall to settle in a vertical column of anticoagulated blood in 1 hour. The Westergren method is the gold standard technique used now.

CRP is another inflammatory marker, a pattern recognition receptor, a key component of the innate immune system, and a member of the pentraxin family with a cyclic pentamer configuration. It was "discovered 70 years ago in the blood of patients with pneumococcal pneumonia" and "reacts with the C-polysaccharide of the pneumococcal bacterial cell wall, hence its name."[30] Analogous to the interaction of antibody with antigen, CRP binds the repeating bacterial polysaccharides and activates the classical complement pathway. In this process, C4 and C3 fragments deposit on bacteria. Adherence and phagocytosis are thereby facilitated.[31-33]

CRP not only increases in response to many inflammatory conditions but also "rapidly decreases with resolution of the process," making it, along with ESR, the 2 most commonly used laboratory tests "to monitor the inflammatory response, particularly in response to treatment."[31]

Literature comparing the ESR with the CRP is limited. ESR is the more commonly used test and has been studied more. However, age, gender, some drugs, and other hematologic factors including anemia affect it. On the other hand, CRP is not affected by these factors and "quantitation is precise and reproducible."[5] In addition, CRP can be stored for sometime and does not require as fresh a serum sample as ESR. Nevertheless, many dispute the true clinical relevance advantages, citing both the additional expense and the increased difficulty of smaller, local laboratories performing the test for such minimal gain.[34]

ESR and CRP are better at following a disease course than at discriminating the presence or absence of the disease in an undifferentiated presentation of joint pain. For example, many people with active RA have normal values of ESR/CRP and many patients with inactive RA have an elevated ESR and/or CRP.[34] Another example is septic arthritis, in which ESR is poor at ruling in or ruling out the disease, with an LR+ = 0.84 (95% CI, 0.60–1.2) and an LR– = 2.4 (95% CI, 0.07–0.89).[26] Furthermore, the acute-phase reactants are not perfect at ruling out temporal arteritis or PMR. Traditionally, the diagnosis of PMR is supported by an ESR greater than 100 mm/h. However, this degree of elevation is "no longer regarded as a sine qua non of these disorders; continuing reports suggest that 10% to 20% of patients with PMR can have 'normal' ESRs ... they have the same frequency of positive temporal artery biopsy results, however, as patients with elevated ESR [69] [70]."[5]

To conclude, ESR and CRP have a final role in evaluating a patient with undifferentiated joint pain, keeping in mind that a normal result cannot rule out disease or discriminate between OA, RA, systemic lupus erythematosus (SLE), or other inflammatory arthropathies. "A more appropriate application of these tests in RA is for monitoring disease activity and response to therapy."[5]

RF

RA is the "most common autoimmune disease, affecting approximately 1% of the world's population."[35,36] Untreated, it is the source of much functional disability primarily from pain, synovitis, and joint destruction. However, because irreversible joint destruction "can be prevented by intervention during the first months of disease, early diagnosis of rheumatoid arthritis is important."[35,37–39]

RF is an IgM autoantibody directed against "antigenic determinants on the crystalizable (F_c) portion of IgG molecules."[5,40] As a laboratory test, RF has both low sensitivity and low specificity. Although it is traditionally associated specifically with RA, many other conditions feature the presence of RF, including lupus, scleroderma, and Sjögren syndrome, as well as tuberculosis, mononucleosis, hepatitis, sarcoidosis, and even chronic obstructive pulmonary disease.[41] In addition, RF may be found in up to 5% to 40% of healthy individuals[42] with the prevalence increasing with age up to 70 to 80 years,[43] when the prevalence decreases possibly because of increasing mortality in seropositive individuals.[5]

Furthermore, RF is only found in approximately 70% of RA patients.[42] Thus, 30% of RA patients are seronegative for RF, and "this proportion can exceed 50% in the early phase of the disease."[44] Nevertheless, the presence of RF is "statistically correlated with a worse prognosis, since higher levels of RF are associated with the presence of aggressive disease, rheumatoid nodules, and extra-articular manifestations."[42]

Therefore, RF in isolation has limited diagnostic value because a negative result for RF does not exclude RA and a positive result should be "carefully interpreted according to the clinical findings."[42–44]

Anti-Cyclic Citrullinated Peptide Antibody

Various other antibodies and serologic markers have been and are being investigated as potential markers of RA activity. Most have been of uncertain clinical benefit in modern clinical practice, with the exception of antibodies to antigens of the anti–cyclic citrullinated peptide (anti-CCP).[42]

Anti-CCP determination has a high sensitivity (70%–75%) and specificity (up to 99%) for RA and is "particularly useful in RF-negative arthritis patients in the early phase of the disease."[42,45]

Measurement of anti-CCP can greatly assist in the workup of early, undifferentiated arthritis and "can increase the prognostic significance of RF."[42,46]

Pathophysiologically, the antibody to anti-CCP is "present before symptoms develop, which suggests that citrullination and production of anti-CCP antibody are early processes in rheumatoid arthritis"[35,46] and seems to be a marker for "more erosive disease" and "poorer functional outcome" even in the absence of RF.[5]

Table 5
Positive and negative likelihood ratios, sensitivity, and specificity (with 95% CI) of anti-CCP compared with RF in predicting RA

	Anti-CCP	RF
Positive Likelihood Ratio	12.46 (9.72–15.98)	4.86 (3.95–5.97)
Negative Likelihood Ratio	0.36 (0.31–0.42)	0.38 (0.33–0.44)
Sensitivity	67% (65%–68%)	95% (95%–96%)
Specificity	69% (68%–70%)	85% (84%–86%)

Data from Nishimura K, Sugiyama D, Kogata Y, et al. Meta-analysis: diagnostic accuracy of anti-cyclic citrullinated peptide antibody and rheumatoid factor for rheumatoid arthritis. Ann Intern Med 2007;146:797–808.

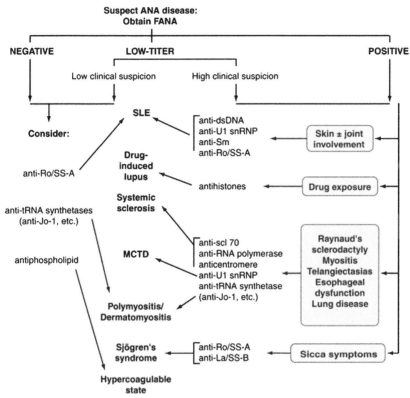

Fig. 1. Algorithm for the use of ANAs in the diagnosis of connective tissue disorders. See text for details. FANA, fluorescent antinuclear antibody test; MCTD, mixed connective tissue disease. (*Modified from* Peng SL, Craft J. Antinuclear antibodies. In: Harris ED, Budd RC, Firestein GS, et al, editors. Kelley's textbook of rheumatology. Philadelphia: W.B. Saunders; 2005. p. 311–31; with permission.)

Table 6		
Incidence and prevalence of selected rheumatologic diseases		
	Incidence in the United States (per 100,000)	Prevalence in the United States (per 100,000)
OA	143	9600
RA	44.6	600
Gout	62.3	2600
Septic Arthritis	n/a	n/a
Lupus (SLE)	5.56	53.6
Scleroderma/CREST Syndrome	1.9	24
Sjögren Syndrome	N/I	N/I
Myositis (polymyositis/ dermatomyositis)	1.8	5.1
PMR	54.8	739
Temporal arteritis	17.8	278

Data from Refs.[27,28,53–55]

Table 7
Sensitivity and specificity of selected rheumatologic illnesses

	Sensitivity	Specificity	NPV	PPV	Likelihood Ratio	Comments
History/Physical Examination						
OA (knee) with at least 3 criteria	0.95	0.69	0.99	0.25	3.06	American College of Rheumatology of OA of the knee clinical criteria are as follows: age >50 y, stiffness <30 min, crepitus, bony tenderness, bony enlargement, and no palpable warmth
OA (knee) with at least 4 clinical criteria	0.84	0.89	0.98	0.48	7.64	
RA					No information available	
Gout	0.98 (0.95–1.02)	0.23 (0.10–0.35)	1.00	0.03	1.27 (1.08–1.50)	Painful joint, swelling, abrupt onset, remission in 2 wk
PMR					No information available	
Temporal arteritis					No information available	
Lupus (SLE)					No information available	
Scleroderma/CREST syndrome					No information available	
Sjögren syndrome					No information available	
Myositis (polymyositis/dermatomyositis)					No information available	
Arthrocentesis						
Septic arthritis (jWBC >50)	0.5 (0.21–0.79)	0.88 (0.8–0.93)			LR+, 4.0 (1.9–8.6); LR−, 0.57 (0.32–1.0)	jWBCs >50,000 cells/mm^3 was considered high
Septic arthritis (jWBC >17.5)	0.83 (0.52–0.98)	0.67 (0.57–0.75)			LR+, 2.5 (1.8–3.6); LR−, 0.25 (0.07–0.89)	jWBCs >17,500 cells/mm^3 was considered high
Gout (urate crystals in acute gout)	0.84 (0.77–0.92)	1 (0.99–1.00)	1.00	1.00	566.6 (35.46–9053.50)	

			No information available			
Gout (urate crystals in intercritical gout)	0.7 (0.50–0.87)	0.95 (0.83–1.08)			15.13 (0.99–229.95)	
RA						
Radiographs						
OA (hip)	0.89	0.9	0.99	0.49	8.9	Osteophytes seen on radiograph of the hip
OA (knee)	0.83	0.93	0.98	0.58	11.86	Knee pain plus osteophytes seen on radiograph of the knee
RA	0.55	0.98	0.98	0.14	27.5	Bone erosions in metacarpal heads and phalangeal bases seen on conventional radiography
RA	0.14	0.99	0.99	0.08	14	Bone erosions in the wrist seen on conventional radiography
Gout (asymmetric swelling seen on radiography)	0.42 (0.33–0.51)	0.9 (0.87–0.92)	0.98	0.10	4.13 (2.97–5.74)	
Gout (subcortical cysts, no erosion)	0.12 (0.06–0.18)	0.98 (0.97–0.99)	0.98	0.14	6.39(3.00–13.57)	
Gout grade II	0.95 (0.86–1.24)	0.07 (–0.01 to 0.15)	0.98	0.03	1.03 (0.90–1.16)	Grade II = tophaceous deposits, eccentric or asymmetric nodular soft tissue masses with or without calcifications (data are from 9 patients)
Gout grade III	0.86 (0.71–1.01)	0.23 (0.09–0.35)	0.98	0.03	1.10 (0.87–1.40)	Grade III = cartilaginous and osseous destruction or grade II findings plus intra-articular or extra-articular erosions of bone and/or joint space narrowing
Gout grade IV	0.57 (0.36–0.78)	0.93 (0.85–1.01)	0.99	0.18	8.00 (2.53–25.31)	Grade IV = grade III findings plus intraosseous calcific deposits, subperiosteal apposition of bone, or bony ankylosis

(continued on next page)

Table 7
(continued)

	Sensitivity	Specificity	NPV	PPV	Likelihood Ratio	Comments
Uric Acid (serum)						
Gout (SUA >6)	0.67 (0.47–0.87)	0.78 (0.51–1.05)	0.99	0.08	3 (0.85–10.57)	
RF						
RA	0.95 (0.95–0.96)	0.85 (0.84–0.86)			LR+, 4.86 (3.95–5.97); LR−, 0.38 (0.33–0.44)	
Anti-CCP						
RA	0.67 (0.65–0.68)	0.69 (0.68–0.70)			LR+, 12.46 (9.72–15.98); LR−, 0.36 (0.31–0.42)	
ANA						
RA	0.41	0.56	0.99	0.01	LR+, 0.93; LR−, 1.06	ANA titers of at least 1:160
Lupus (SLE)	0.93	0.57	0.99	0.00	LR+, 2.2; LR−, 0.11	
Scleroderma/CREST syndrome	0.85	0.54	1.00	0.00	LR+, 1.86; LR−, 0.27	
Sjögren syndrome	0.48	0.52	0.99	0.14	LR+, 0.99; LR−, 1.01	
Myositis (polymyositis/dermatomyositis)	0.61	0.63	1.00	0.00	LR+, 1.67; LR−, 0.61	

Abbreviations: JWBC, white blood cells in joint fluid; SUA, serum uric acid.
Data from Refs.[25,26,56–59]

Furthermore, levels of anti-CCP antibodies are detected early in the course of RA and increase throughout the disease process; the antibodies function as useful "markers of the progression and prognosis of the disease."[42,46]

Table 5 summarizes the positive and negative likelihood ratios, sensitivity, and specificity (with 95% CI) of anti-CCP compared with the RF from a recent large meta-analysis.[35]

So which antibody should be used: the RF or the anti-CCP? Some have proposed that if a patient's clinical likelihood of RA is low based on interview, examination, and ACR criteria, measuring anti-CCP antibody without the RF seems to avoid too many false positives.[35] This strategy, especially when applied in the lower-likelihood context of a primary care clinic, can avoid the potential harm and expense of treating anti-CCP antibody–negative and RF-positive individuals. However, further clinical trials and cost-effective studies of these trade-offs are needed.[35] Because RF is still included in the 1987 ACR criteria, it remains a recommended screening test for RA, and both tests together maximize sensitivity.[35,47]

Antinuclear Antibodies

Antinuclear antibodies (ANAs)—and many other measurable antibodies against other cytoplasmic entities—play a key role in the pathogenesis and diagnosis of many auto-immune diseases and are found in diseases such as SLE, systemic sclerosis, inflammatory myositis, and Sjögren syndrome.[1] A negative titer to ANAs does not rule out many of the conditions being sought by ordering the test.[48] Also, although ANAs are useful and even essential diagnostic laboratory tests for these diseases, up to 20% to 31% of healthy volunteer blood donors were found to be seropositive for ANAs.[5,48–50] In addition, other less characteristic diseases sometimes feature sero-positivity to ANAs, such as autoimmune hepatitis, primary biliary cirrhosis, idiopathic thrombocytopenic purpura (ITP), and multiple sclerosis. Thus, "positive ANA tests are much more prevalent than connective tissue diseases," especially in the elderly, and "most of the abnormal results are falsely positive."[48]

The ANA titer has some discriminating power. For example, 20% to 30% of healthy, disease-free individuals have an ANA titer greater than or equal to 1:40.[5,51] Thus, this range is frequently quoted as the threshold of abnormal by most laboratories, although up to 12% of normal individuals may have a titer greater than or equal to 1:80.[5,51] ANA titers as high as 1:640 can be seen in children who do not have SLE.[52]

Like the other laboratory modalities discussed, the ANA test should only be ordered in the context of clinical signs that correlate with related diseases. ANA testing is particularly helpful for 4 primary conditions, when suspected: SLE, systemic sclerosis (scleroderma), polymyositis/dermatomyositis, and Sjögren syndrome.[5,51]

In addition to diagnostic value, there exist diseases in which the ANA may have a prognostic value (eg, juvenile RA, antiphospholipid antibody syndrome, and Raynaud phenomenon).[5,48,51] Conversely, other diseases feature a significant number of individuals that are ANA positive, but this has little diagnostic or prognostic power (eg, RA, 30%–50%; fibromyalgia, 15%–25%; ITP, 10%–30%; and multiple sclerosis, 25%,).

Measurement of individual ANA can also be performed, but typically, it should be measured "only in the context of clinical signs that correlate with antibody-disease associations (e.g., anti-DNA or anti-Sm in the suspicion of systemic lupus erythematosus)." A useful algorithm to navigate the complicated array of individual ANAs is seen in **Fig. 1**.[1]

Other Miscellaneous Tests

Although many other tests exist to help elucidate in the right clinical circumstance, 3 other specific tests may have more of a first-line status. Firstly, patients with tuberculosis can have, or even present with, monoarthritis. Vigilance during the history and review of systems is critical to alert the clinician to the need to order acid-fast bacillus smear and culture on arthrocentesis, as well as skin testing (Mantoux or PPD).

Secondly, serum anti-Borrelia titers can be useful in areas and/or circumstances where the likelihood of Lyme disease is substantial, and when negative, Lyme disease is unlikely. Like any test, false positives confound broad application of this test. Finally, antistreptolysin O is a useful test in the setting of undifferentiated arthritis when known or suspected recent streptococcal exposure has occurred. When negative, rheumatic fever is highly unlikely.

SUMMARY

"In evaluating patients for systemic autoimmune disease, however, advances in diagnostic testing have not supplanted a carefully performed history and physical examination. In fact, many common rheumatologic conditions, including bursitis, tendinitis, fibromyalgia, and osteoarthritis, can be reliably diagnosed without any confirmatory laboratory or imaging tests."[48] Conversely, in clinical practice, an individual laboratory test is "insufficient to establish or refute" most important rheumatologic diagnoses.[5] Thus, although laboratory testing is important, history, physical examination, and clinical context retain their primacy. **Tables 6** and **7** offer information regarding the sensitivity, specificity, and prevalence of selected rheumatologic diseases to assist in selecting the correct diagnostic cascade.

ACKNOWLEDGMENTS

The author acknowledges the research contribution of Saman Razzak, MD, to **Tables 6** and **7**; thanks Nelle Williams and Sharon Glenn of the Health Sciences Library; and acknowledges the administrative support of Stephanie Beers and Alison Adams.

REFERENCES

1. Palmer T, Toombs JD. Managing joint pain in primary care. J Am Board Fam Pract 2004;17(Suppl):S32–42.
2. Phillips A, Polisson R. The rational initial clinical evaluation of the patient with musculoskeletal complaints. Am J Med 1997;103:7S–11S.
3. Alarcón G, Willkens R, Ward J, et al. Early undifferentiated connective tissue disease. IV. Musculoskeletal manifestations in a large cohort of patients with undifferentiated connective tissue diseases compared with cohorts of patients with well-established connective tissue diseases: followup analyses in patients with unexplained polyarthritis and patients with rheumatoid arthritis at baseline. Arthritis Rheum 1996;39:403–14.
4. Shmerling R, Delbanco T. The rheumatoid factor: an analysis of clinical utility. Am J Med 1991;91:528–34.
5. Firestein GS, Budd RC, Harris ED Jr, et al. Kelley's textbook of rheumatology. 8th edition. Philadelphia: W.B. Saunders; 2008.
6. Jaeschke R, Guyatt G, Sackett DL. Users' guides to the medical literature. III. How to use an article about a diagnostic test. A. Are the results of the study valid? Evidence-Based Medicine Working Group. JAMA 1994;271:389–91.

7. Jaeschke R, Guyatt GH, Sackett DL. Users' guides to the medical literature. III. How to use an article about a diagnostic test. B. What are the results and will they help me in caring for my patients? The Evidence-Based Medicine Working Group. JAMA 1994;271:703–7.

8. LLC. Prevention: epidemiology. 2008. Family Practice Notebook; 2010. Available at: http://www.fpnotebook.com/Prevent/Epi/index.htm. Accessed June 28, 2010.

9. Waits JB. SpIn and SnOut. 2010. Available at: http://tinyurl.com/SensSpec. Accessed June 28, 2010.

10. Thomsen T, Shen S, Shaffer R, et al. Videos in clinical medicine. Arthrocentesis of the knee. N Engl J Med 2006;354:e19.

11. Siva C, Velazquez C, Mody A, et al. Diagnosing acute monoarthritis in adults: a practical approach for the family physician. Am Fam Physician 2003;68:83–90.

12. John P, Michael T, Grant F, et al. Pfenninger and Fowler's procedures for primary care 2nd edition and multimedia primary care procedures. St Louis (MO): Saunders; 2005.

13. Zuber T. Knee joint aspiration and injection. Am Fam Physician 2002;66: 1497–500, 503–504, 507.

14. McGinn TG, Guyatt GH, Wyer PC, et al. Users' guides to the medical literature: XXII: how to use articles about clinical decision rules. Evidence-Based Medicine Working Group. JAMA 2000;284:79–84.

15. Stiell IG, McKnight RD, Greenberg GH, et al. Implementation of the Ottawa Ankle Rules. JAMA 1994;271:827–32.

16. Stiell IG, Wells GA, Hoag RH, et al. Implementation of the Ottawa Knee Rule for the use of radiography in acute knee injuries. JAMA 1997;278:2075–9.

17. Ottawa Hospital Research Institute, Ottawa Ankle Rules. 2005. Available at: http://www.ohri.ca/emerg/cdr/ankle.html. Accessed June 28, 2010.

18. Jacobson JA, Daffner RH, Weissman BN, et al, for Expert Panel on Musculoskeletal Imaging. ACR Appropriateness Criteria® chronic ankle pain. Reston (VA): American College of Radiology (ACR); 2009. p. 8 [online].

19. Jacobson JA, Daffner RH, Weissman BN, et al, for Expert Panel on Musculoskeletal Imaging. ACR Appropriateness Criteria® chronic elbow pain. Reston (VA): American College of Radiology (ACR); 2008. p. 8 [online].

20. Wise JN, Daffner RH, Weissman BN, et al, for Expert Panel on Musculoskeletal Imaging. ACR Appropriateness Criteria® chronic foot pain. Reston (VA): American College of Radiology (ACR); 2008. p. 8 [online].

21. Taljanovic M, Daffner RH, Weissman BN, et al, for Expert Panel on Musculoskeletal Imaging. ACR Appropriateness Criteria® chronic hip pain. Reston (VA): American College of Radiology (ACR); 2008. p. 8 [online].

22. Daffner RH, Weissman BN, Bennett DL, et al, for Expert Panel on Musculoskeletal Imaging. ACR Appropriateness Criteria® chronic neck pain. Reston (VA): American College of Radiology (ACR); 2008. p. 7 [online].

23. Blebea JS, Lott KE, Weissman BN, et al, for Expert Panel on Musculoskeletal Imaging. ACR Appropriateness Criteria® chronic wrist pain. Reston (VA): American College of Radiology (ACR); 2009. p. 9 [online].

24. Bennett DL, Daffner RH, Weissman BN, et al, for Expert Panel on Musculoskeletal Imaging. ACR Appropriateness Criteria® chronic knee pain. Reston (VA): American College of Radiology (ACR); 2008. p. 7 [online].

25. Cibere J. Do we need radiographs to diagnose osteoarthritis? Best Pract Res Clin Rheumatol 2006;20:27–38.

26. Li SF, Cassidy C, Chang C, et al. Diagnostic utility of laboratory tests in septic arthritis. Emerg Med J 2007;24:75–7.

27. Lawrence RC, Felson DT, Helmick CG, et al. Estimates of the prevalence of arthritis and other rheumatic conditions in the United States. Part II. Arthritis Rheum 2008;58:26–35.
28. Helmick CG, Felson DT, Lawrence RC, et al. Estimates of the prevalence of arthritis and other rheumatic conditions in the United States. Part I. Arthritis Rheum 2008;58:15–25.
29. Campion E, Glynn R, DeLabry L. Asymptomatic hyperuricemia. Risks and consequences in the Normative Aging Study. Am J Med 1987;82:421–6.
30. Mold C, Nakayama S, Holzer T, et al. C-reactive protein is protective against Streptococcus pneumoniae infection in mice. J Exp Med 1981; 154:1703–8.
31. Atkinson JP. C-reactive protein: a rheumatologist's friend revisited. Arthritis Rheum 2001;44:995–6.
32. Gabay C, Kushner I. Acute-phase proteins and other systemic responses to inflammation. N Engl J Med 1999;340:448–54.
33. Du Clos T. Function of C-reactive protein. Ann Med 2000;32:274–8.
34. Wolfe F. The many myths of erythrocyte sedimentation rate and C-reactive protein. J Rheumatol 2009;36:1568–9.
35. Nishimura K, Sugiyama D, Kogata Y, et al. Meta-analysis: diagnostic accuracy of anti-cyclic citrullinated peptide antibody and rheumatoid factor for rheumatoid arthritis. Ann Intern Med 2007;146:797–808.
36. Lee D, Weinblatt M. Rheumatoid arthritis. Lancet 2001;358:903–11.
37. Landewé R. The benefits of early treatment in rheumatoid arthritis: confounding by indication, and the issue of timing. Arthritis Rheum 2003;48:1–5.
38. Lard L, Visser H, Speyer I, et al. Early versus delayed treatment in patients with recent-onset rheumatoid arthritis: comparison of two cohorts who received different treatment strategies. Am J Med 2001;111:446–51.
39. Bukhari M, Wiles N, Lunt M, et al. Influence of disease-modifying therapy on radiographic outcome in inflammatory polyarthritis at five years: results from a large observational inception study. Arthritis Rheum 2003;48:46–53.
40. Renaudineau Y, Jamin C, Saraux A, et al. Rheumatoid factor on a daily basis. Autoimmunity 2005;38:11–6.
41. Wolfe F, Cathey M, Roberts F. The latex test revisited. Rheumatoid factor testing in 8,287 rheumatic disease patients. Arthritis Rheum 1991;34:951–60.
42. da Mota LM, dos Santos Neto LL, de Carvalho JF. Autoantibodies and other serological markers in rheumatoid arthritis: predictors of disease activity? Clin Rheumatol 2009;28:1127–34.
43. Visser H, Gelinck L, Kampfraath A, et al. Diagnostic and prognostic characteristics of the enzyme linked immunosorbent rheumatoid factor assays in rheumatoid arthritis. Ann Rheum Dis 1996;55:157–61.
44. Visser H. Early diagnosis of rheumatoid arthritis. Best Pract Res Clin Rheumatol 2005;19:55–72.
45. Raza K, Breese M, Nightingale P, et al. Predictive value of antibodies to cyclic citrullinated peptide in patients with very early inflammatory arthritis. J Rheumatol 2005;32:231–8.
46. Rantapää-Dahlqvist S, de Jong B, Berglin E, et al. Antibodies against cyclic citrullinated peptide and IgA rheumatoid factor predict the development of rheumatoid arthritis. Arthritis Rheum 2003;48:2741–9.
47. Wiik A, Gordon T, Kavanaugh A, et al. Cutting edge diagnostics in rheumatology: the role of patients, clinicians, and laboratory scientists in optimizing the use of autoimmune serology. Arthritis Rheum 2004;51:291–8.

48. Blumenthal DE. Tired, aching, ANA-positive: does your patient have lupus or fibromyalgia? Cleve Clin J Med 2002;69:143–6, 51–2.
49. de Vlam K, De Keyser F, Verbruggen G, et al. Detection and identification of antinuclear autoantibodies in the serum of normal blood donors. Clin Exp Rheumatol 1993;11:393–7.
50. Craig W, Ledue T, Johnson A, et al. The distribution of antinuclear antibody titers in "normal" children and adults. J Rheumatol 1999;26:914–9.
51. Kavanaugh A, Tomar R, Reveille J, et al. Guidelines for clinical use of the antinuclear antibody test and tests for specific autoantibodies to nuclear antigens. American College of Pathologists. Arch Pathol Lab Med 2000;124:71–81.
52. McGhee JL, Kickingbird LM, Jarvis JN. Clinical utility of antinuclear antibody tests in children. BMC Pediatr 2004;4:13.
53. Doran MF, Pond GR, Crowson CS, et al. Trends in incidence and mortality in rheumatoid arthritis in Rochester, Minnesota, over a forty-year period. Arthritis Rheum 2002;46:625–31.
54. Mayes MD. Scleroderma epidemiology. Rheum Dis Clin North Am 2003;29: 239–54.
55. Jacobson D, Gange S, Rose N, et al. Epidemiology and estimated population burden of selected autoimmune diseases in the United States. Clin Immunol Immunopathol 1997;84:223–43.
56. Jackson JL, O'Malley PG, Kroenke K. Evaluation of acute knee pain in primary care. Ann Intern Med 2003;139:575–88.
57. Zhang W, Doherty M, Pascual E, et al. EULAR evidence based recommendations for gout. Part I: diagnosis. Report of a task force of the Standing Committee for International Clinical Studies Including Therapeutics (ESCISIT). Ann Rheum Dis 2006;65:1301–11.
58. Duer-Jensen A, Vestergaard A, Dohn UM, et al. Detection of rheumatoid arthritis bone erosions by two different dedicated extremity MRI units and conventional radiography. Ann Rheum Dis 2008;67:998–1003.
59. Habash-Bseiso DE, Yale SH, Glurich I, et al. Serologic testing in connective tissue diseases. Clin Med Res 2005;3:190–3.

Arthrocentesis and Therapeutic Joint Injection: An Overview for the Primary Care Physician

R. Brian Bettencourt, MD*, Michael M. Linder, MD

KEYWORDS

• Arthrocentesis • Joint • Effusion • Steroid • Injection

Arthrocentesis is a safe and useful primary care procedure. Joint aspiration and injection can be both diagnostic and therapeutic; it can allow identification and treatment of pathologic agents as well as provide significant pain relief. There are numerous conditions affecting adults and children that may lead to mono- or polyarticular joint swelling. Causes can range from rheumatic to infectious to idiopathic, and thorough investigations of each may require specific serologic studies or specialist consultation. This review provides current and practical recommendations for evaluation and localized treatment of effusive joint pain by the primary care physician.

INDICATIONS AND CLINICAL EVIDENCE

Multiple indications exist for arthrocentesis. Synovial fluid aspiration may be indicated in any joint with an effusion, or even in a normal-appearing joint when the diagnosis is in doubt. There are many causes for joint effusions in adults and children (**Table 1**). When evaluating a synovial effusion of unknown origin, aspiration is indicated.[1] Arthrocentesis is essential for the diagnosis and management of the acute hot red joint, which may be a medical emergency secondary to the morbidity and mortality associated with septic arthritis.[2]

With or without subsequent therapeutic injection, arthrocentesis of a joint effusion can often provide pain relief. Traumatic injury to a joint may cause hemarthrosis and effusions ranging from small to large, tense and painful. Aspiration of large traumatic effusions can ease pain and allow for increased range of motion.

The authors have nothing to disclose.
Family Medicine Residency Program, University of South Alabama, 1504 Springhill Avenue, Room 3414, Mobile, AL 36604, USA
* Corresponding author.
E-mail address: rbettencourt@usouthal.edu

Prim Care Clin Office Pract 37 (2010) 691–702
doi:10.1016/j.pop.2010.07.002
0095-4543/10/$ – see front matter © 2010 Published by Elsevier Inc.

Table 1	
Differential of an acute joint with effusion	
Infectious	Osteoarthritis
Bacterial	Rheumatologic
Viral	Rheumatoid arthritis
Lyme disease	Juvenile idiopathic arthritis
Bacterial endocarditis sequelae	Systemic lupus erythematosus
Crystalline disease	Spondyloarthropathy
Gout	Transient synovitis
Pseudogout (CPPD)	Systemic vasculitis
Hydroxyapatite	Neoplastic
Hemarthrosis	Pigmented villonodular synovitis
Coagulopathy	Metastatic disease
Trauma	Idiopathic

Data from Refs.[1,2,27,28,32–38]

CONTRAINDICATIONS

Diagnostic arthrocentesis has few contraindications. Periarticular cellulitis or infection is considered an absolute contraindication to joint aspiration. The concern is that the joint might be seeded by organisms of the overlying skin infection during percutaneous access. However, if the joint is believed to be the cause of the infection, diagnostic aspiration should be performed. The attempt should be made through an area of appropriately prepared uninvolved skin. Joint access through an area of irregular or disrupted skin, such as in psoriasis, should be avoided because of increased numbers of colonizing bacteria in these areas.[3]

Septicemia has been considered a contraindication to arthrocentesis secondary to the possibility of introducing organisms into the joint space. The morbidity and mortality associated with a septic joint are substantial. Joints with a high suspicion for bacterial infection should probably undergo aspiration regardless of the presence of septicemia. Septicemia may be the initial finding in young children with bacterial arthritis. The risk of leaving a septic joint improperly treated seems to outweigh the theoretic risk of seeding.

In patients with bleeding disorders or who are taking anticoagulants, joint aspiration is contraindicated. Inducing traumatic hemarthrosis is a concern. However, the risk of significant hemarthrosis after arthrocentesis is low. At least 1 study showed that even in patients on warfarin therapy with international normalized ratios of 4.5, there was not an increased risk of significant bleeding.[4]

COMPLICATIONS OF ARTHROCENTESIS

Generally, the most feared complication of arthrocentesis is iatrogenic infection. Although there is a lack of recent large studies, iatrogenic infection after arthrocentesis seems rare but remains a possible complication. In studies in which injection sites were stained before percutaneous needle access of a joint, investigators were able to arthroscopically identify transferred fragments of the stained skin within the joint in most cases.[5] Although iatrogenic infection seems rare, these findings serve to reinforce the importance of sound aseptic technique and skin preparation during the procedure.

SYNOVIAL FLUID AND EFFUSIONS

There are numerous causes for joint effusions. The gross appearance of synovial fluid can provide clues related to the type and degree of joint pathology.

Historically, 1 step in clinical diagnosis has been to assign results of synovial fluid visual inspection to 1 of 5 categories: normal, inflammatory, noninflammatory, hemorrhagic, or septic (**Table 2**). Each category can have an association with a specific disease process.

On visual inspection, inflammatory-appearing fluid may suggest crystalline joint disease or any number of rheumatologic conditions. Noninflammatory appearing fluid may be present in joints with osteoarthritis. It is important to remember during clinical decision making that there can be significant overlap between categories.

Normal synovial fluid is clear, colorless to pale yellow, and highly viscous. Fluid of an inflammatory source ranges from yellow to greenish yellow and may be white in the crystalline arthropathies (eg, gout, calcium pyrophosphate dehydrate [CPPD]). Septic joints can yield greenish, gray, or purulent fluid. Red, rusty, or brownish fluid suggests hemarthrosis. The viscosity and turbidity of synovial fluid varies with the cause. Turbidity can be expected to increase with the degree of inflammation.[3]

Viscosity can be variable. The "string sign" has been used as a subjective examination whereby normally viscous fluid dripped out of a syringe stretches to 3 cm in length before breaking. Inflammation with release of proteolytic enzymes generally decreases synovial fluid viscosity. However, septic fluid may show increasing viscosity with increased purulence.

LABORATORY ANALYSIS OF SYNOVIAL FLUID

Laboratory analysis of synovial fluid is the single most important assessment technique when investigating an effusion of unclear etiology. It is essential in any investigation of a suspected septic joint. Synovial fluid analysis also allows for diagnosis of specific crystalline arthropathies, and helps to determine whether the cause may be inflammatory or noninflammatory.

For formal study, collected synovial fluid can be divided into 4 aliquots. One of the 4 should be a sterile tube with anticoagulant for bacteriologic studies. One tube with eth-ylenediaminetetraacetic acid should be sent for routine cytology, and another tube without anticoagulant should be prepared for crystal search and analysis. The remaining fluid may be reserved for other specialized studies if indicated.[5]

Often the volume of available fluid for study may be limited. Ruling out a septic etiology is the primary concern when evaluating an effused joint. In such cases, laboratory analysis of synovial fluid should include a white blood cell (WBC) count with differential, Gram stain, and culture.

CYTOLOGY

Normal synovial fluid should be nearly free of cells. Samples indicating an inflammatory cause show increasing numbers of leukocytes, with the WBC cutoff of 2000 cells/μL generally accepted as distinguishing noninflammatory from inflammatory

Table 2
Gross visual inspection of synovial fluid aspirate

	Normal	Noninflammatory	Inflammatory	Infectious	Hemorrhagic
Appearance	Clear to pale yellow	Clear, yellow	Cloudy, yellow	Purulent or cloudy	Bloody
Viscosity	High	High	Low	Variable	Variable

Data from Refs.[1,2,27,28,32–38]

conditions. The widely accepted WBC count defining septic synovial fluid has classically been greater than 50,000 WBC/µL.[6] However, in one recent study of culture-positive synovial fluid aspirates, 39% had synovial WBC counts of less than 50,000 cells/µL.[7] Another similar study found greatly increased likelihood for septic arthritis with synovial WBC counts equal to or greater than 25,000 cells/µL, but a polymorphonuclear leukocyte count less than 90% significantly decreased the likelihood of a septic cause. Thus 25,000 cells/µL may be a more accurate threshold if there is concern regarding septic arthritis.[8]

Additional information regarding synovial fluid findings can be found in **Table 3**.

CRYSTAL DETECTION

Synovial fluid analysis is useful in establishing a diagnosis of crystal-induced arthritis. The CPPD of pseudogout appear as positively birefringent rhomboid crystals under polarized microscopy. Definitive diagnosis of CPPD generally requires the addition of characteristic joint findings on imaging. The monosodium urate crystals of gout are negatively birefringent under polarized light microscopy, and their presence is diagnostic of gout.

GRAM STAIN AND CULTURE

Studies to evaluate for microbes are essential in the evaluation of an effusion of unknown cause. The sensitivity of the Gram stain in bacterial arthritis is generally 50% to 70%, with the exception being gonococcal arthritis (perhaps <10%).[9,10] Cultures are generally positive in most cases of bacterial arthritis, the exception again being gonococcal arthritis (<50%).[11,12] Even in joint aspirates from patients with confirmed crystal-induced arthritis, one study reported that 1.5% had concomitant synovial bacterial infections.[13] In the setting of an unexplained joint effusion the synovial fluid investigation should include Gram stain and culture even if the fluid appears inflammatory.

Table 3
Synovial fluid analysis

	Normal	Noninflammatory	Inflammatory	Infectious
Culture	Negative	Negative	Negative	Often positive
WBC/µL	<200	<200–2000	200–50,000	>25,000–50,000
Polymorphonuclear leukocytes (%)	<25	<25	>50	>50–90
Crystals	Negative	Negative	Positive or none	None
Associated conditions		Osteoarthritis	Rheumatic diseases, crystalline diseases, spondyloarthropathies, systemic lupus erythematosus	Septic arthritis

Data from Refs.[1,2,3,6–8,27,28,32–38]

BACTERIAL ARTHRITIS

Intraarticular corticosteroid injection is contraindicated in cases of suspected bacterial arthritis. Corticosteroids inhibit the ability of the immune system to fight off infection. The patient with septic arthritis generally requires inpatient care with intravenous antibiotics and orthopedic specialist consultation. Specifics and management are discussed elsewhere in this issue.

INJECTION IN INFLAMMATORY ARTHRITIS

Intraarticular corticosteroids injections are commonly used to treat inflammatory joint conditions such as the rheumatoid and crystal-induced arthropathies. Much of the experience in this area has been with conditions such as rheumatoid arthritis, juvenile idiopathic arthritis, psoriatic arthritis, and reactive arthritis. There are anecdotal reports of use in less common conditions such as sarcoidosis and systemic lupus erythematosus, but there seem to be no large-scale studies using intraarticular steroids in those conditions.

Corticosteroid injections are frequently used in the treatment of rheumatoid arthritis as an adjunct to disease-modifying drug therapy. Several large studies support their efficacy and safety. Removal of joint fluid by aspiration before instilling the steroid has been shown to improve short-term outcomes.[14] Serial injection in inflamed rheumatic joints has been shown to be superior to systemic steroids, to be helpful in obtaining clinical remission, and to reduce radiographic progression of disease.[15,16]

The mainstay of treatment in most crystal-induced arthritis is intervention to control serum uric acid levels and oral analgesia. However, therapeutic injection is an effective treatment of exacerbations. Intraarticular corticosteroids generally lead to faster resolution, and most patients can anticipate relief within 24 to 48 hours of administration.[3]

INJECTION IN NONINFLAMMATORY ARTHRITIS

Osteoarthritis is typified by gradual degeneration of articular cartilage with the development of joint pain, stiffness, and losses in range of motion. The knee is the most commonly affected joint. When standard therapies such as physical therapy and oral analgesics do not provide adequate relief, intraarticular corticosteroids are commonly used to treat pain and swelling associated with osteoarthritis. Generally, in those who show a response, maximum benefit seems to last from 1 to 6 weeks, with waning effect by 12 weeks after injection.[17] As with the treatment of rheumatoid arthritis, there seems to be better response to therapeutic injection if fluid is first aspirated from the joint space.[7]

Hyaluronic acid (HA) derivatives can be used to treat pain associated with osteoarthritis of the knee and have been the subject of much study in recent years. These preparations can be delivered as a single dose or as a series of 3 to 5 weekly injections. Some meta-analysis reviews suggest that HA treatments may have a modest pain relief advantage over oral nonsteroidal anti-inflammatory drugs (NSAIDs). One recent review that compared the efficacy of corticosteroid versus HA over time suggested that steroid injection may give better results from week 0 to week 4, but that an HA showed better efficacy from week 8 to week 26.[18] Choice of therapy is dependent on individual practitioner experience and preference.

CORTICOSTEROID PREPARATIONS

There seems to be no consensus on the type of steroid that is best used for therapeutic joint injection. Commonly used agents are triamcinolone preparations

(Kenalog, Aristospan), methylprednisolone (Depo-Medrol), and betamethasone (Celestone Soluspan). There seems to be significant regional variation in choice of steroid.[19] There is anecdotal evidence that use of betamethasone (Celestone Soluspan) may result in better outcomes (**Box 1**). **Table 4** identifies how much volume of this preparation each joint tolerates.

Current standard practice is to include a volume of local anesthetic during therapeutic injection. This addition can give the patient fast temporary pain relief, and the added fluid volume is believed to help distribute the steroid within the joint. Depending on the size of the joint, between 3 and 7 mL of 1% lidocaine can be included with intraarticular steroid injections.

RISKS AND COMPLICATIONS

Although the incidence is low, iatrogenic infection is considered the primary risk associated with intraarticular injection. Estimates of actual risk vary by an order of magnitude from 1 in 10,000 to 1 in 100,000.[20,21] This risk, as well as warning signs and symptoms, should be included in an informed consent discussion with the patient before the procedure.

Redness and swelling that can be mistaken for signs of infection rarely occur after the procedure. This phenomenon, termed postinjection flare, can have onset a few hours to 2 days after an injection. Believed to be an inflammatory reaction to the steroid crystals themselves, postinjection flare is estimated to occur in 1% to 6% of such therapeutic injections.[3] The effect is self limited and usually responds to application of ice packs. If not contraindicated, oral NSAIDs can be given for a few days to decrease the probability of postinjection flare.[22,23]

There is evidence that local steroid injections may exert some systemic effects. One study documented decreases in plasma cortisol lasting 2 to 7 days after a single injection.[23] However, the degree and duration of adrenal suppression from an intraarticular injection of depot steroid is less than that seen from an equivalent intramuscular

---

Box 1
Steps for combined intraarticular aspiration and injection

1. Discuss risks and benefits with patient and obtain informed consent
2. Prepare equipment and medication
3. Identify and mark appropriate landmarks and/or point of needle placement
4. Clean overlying skin using povidone-iodine (Betadine) or isopropyl alcohol
5. Use cooling spray or local anesthetic for patient comfort (as needed)
6. Select appropriate length and gauge of needle
7. Introduce needle into intraarticular space
8. Gently aspirate fluid
9. Anchor needle with hemostat to prevent migration from the intraarticular space
10. Remove aspirate syringe and replace with syringe containing steroid and/or anesthetic for injection
11. Introduce medication into the intraarticular space
12. Remove needle and apply dressing
13. Provide postprocedural counseling
14. Monitor patient for adverse reactions

Table 4			
Volume of preparation tolerated by joint			
Joint/Area	Betamethasone (mL)	Lidocaine (1%) (mL)	Hydrocortisone Equivalents (mg)
Knee	2–3	5–7	300–450
Shoulder	1–2	5–7	150–300
Subacromial	1–2	5–7	150–300
Elbow	1–2	3–5	150–300

dose.[24,25] Patients who are diabetic should closely monitor their serum glucose measurements for 2 weeks following an intraarticular injection because systemic effects could cause temporary increases. Some patients may experience transient flushing or diaphoresis after procedure. This reaction is presumably secondary to systemic effect or possibly from a reaction to preservatives in the steroid preparation.[3]

There has been discussion regarding steroid-induced cartilaginous arthropathy with frequent injection of the same joint. There is a lack of consensus in the literature regarding frequency of administration, and concerns about corticosteroid-mediated arthropathy persist. Most large studies do not support this as a significant risk in either rheumatoid or osteoarthritis treatment. A prudent approach seems to be applying corticosteroid injection to an individual joint no more than 4 times a year. Although the adjunctive use of a local anesthetic mixed in with the steroid for injection has become standard, recent animal studies have suggested that chondrocyte viability may be adversely affected by exposure to common local anesthetics in a dose-dependent manner.[26,27] There are no human studies at this time but future modifications of this currently common practice may occur as a result.

TECHNIQUE

Injection of the shoulder, elbow, or knee can be considered an adjunctive therapy. Generally, it may be used after other appropriate therapeutic interventions have been undertaken. These interventions include oral pain relievers, physical therapy, and in the case of rheumatoid arthritis should not replace disease-modifying agents.

Arthrocentesis and injection are best performed using sterile surgical gloves and aseptic technique. An 18- to 22-gauge needle should be used for medium to large joints, and a syringe of up to 60 mL volume (or rarely 2 syringes for a large knee effusion) should be available. If possible the patient should be placed in a comfortable supine or upright position. The involved area should be prepared with povidone-iodine (Betadine) and draped. One key to success in accessing a joint space is a solid understanding of the anatomy and associated landmarks of the joint; a quick review is never detrimental.

There are several approaches to skin anesthesia before arthrocentesis. Subcutaneous 1% lidocaine delivered through a high-gauge needle can be used at the point of injection to lessen discomfort. When treating children, pretreatment with topical eutectic lidocaine/prilocaine cream may or may not be effective.[28] Ethyl chloride spray is an excellent option. It is a rapidly evaporating coolant that provides good superficial anesthesia at the point of injection.

Interest in ultrasound guidance during joint aspiration and injection has increased in recent years. It has previously been reported to increase the rate of successful aspiration in joint spaces that are difficult to access. Other investigators have asserted that in most uncomplicated cases the use of standard anatomic landmarks results in correct needle placement. Recent publications support the usefulness of sonographic guidance in large joint aspiration and injection. Studies have shown greater aspirate fluid volume with sonographic needle guidance during arthrocentesis, and there is increasing evidence of intraarticular injection accuracy and decreased procedural pain over anatomic landmark placement.[29]

Aspiration of fluid should be performed before corticosteroid injection, not only to improve therapeutic outcomes as described earlier, but to help verify intraarticular needle placement. Removal of the aspirate syringe and replacement with a syringe with the corticosteroid preparation can be cumbersome. To ensure continued intraarticular placement, and to decrease the amount of needle tip movement, many physicians secure the needle with a hemostat during changeover.

KNEE

The knee is the most commonly and easily aspirated joint. There are many different successful techniques. It may be accessed via a lateral, medial, or anterior approach, with the patient either supine and the joint in nearly full extension, or with the patient sitting upright with the leg dependent and knee in 90° flexion. Many find that a lateral approach is easiest. Position the patient supine in near full knee extension with a rolled towel under the popliteal space for support when attempting this approach. The knee is comprised of 2 functional joints: the femoral-tibial and the femoral-patellar joints. A recess can be palpated approximately 1 to 2 fingerbreadths superior and 1 to 2 fingerbreadths lateral of the superior margin of the lateral patella. The joint can be accessed with a needle through this recess.[22]

Before sterile preparation, identify and mark this area of access using either an indentation in the skin or ink for a guidance mark. After preparation and application of topical anesthesia, an 18- to 22-gauge needle can be directed at a 45° angle distally and 45° into the knee (**Fig. 1**). Advance the needle slowly and purposefully about 1 to 3 cm into the joint space while gently aspirating the syringe.[3] Using a free hand to compress the opposite side of the joint or patella may aid in arthrocentesis.

Care should be taken during the procedure. Striking boney or articular surfaces with a needle can cause patient discomfort. When fluid flows easily into the syringe, stop advancement of the needle and continue smooth constant aspiration. The suprapatellar pouch communicates with the joint space, and extends well above the patella. Fluid aspiration from an effused knee may be further enhanced by applying mild manual

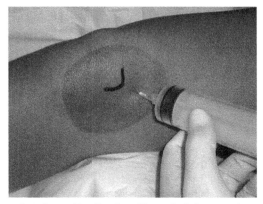

Fig. 1. Lateral approach to knee. Needle placed lateral of the superior margin of the lateral patella (black outline identifies superior lateral border of patella).

pressure and milking fluid down from this space. After changeover from the aspiration syringe to the prepared syringe, the suspension should be introduced slowly and smoothly.

SHOULDER

The glenohumeral joint is the most mobile joint of the body. It is supported by the joint capsule and several ligaments and muscles. Therapeutic injection of the shoulder can be used in treatment of various systemic processes, overuse syndromes, and injuries. A suspected tear in the rotator cuff is a relative contraindication. The glenohumeral joint is a small space and accessing it can prove more challenging than the knee. Landmarks for the procedure include the acromion, the head of the humerus, and the coracoid process.[30]

Fig. 2 shows a posterior approach. The patient is positioned upright with the humerus in a dependent position. Palpation of the posterior area of the shoulder should reveal a recess found 2 to 3 cm below the posterolateral corner of the acromion. The needle is introduced and advanced anteromedially and slightly inferiorly. The tip of the needle should be directed at the coracoid process while the syringe is gently aspirated (**Fig. 2**). Even after a thorough history and physical examination, the exact cause of shoulder pain can remain unclear. For ease and practicality, a therapeutic injection into the subacromial space is often beneficial to nearby structures such as the subdeltoid bursa, subacromial bursa, and rotator cuff tendons.[3]

To access the subacromial space, the needle is inserted just inferior to the posterolateral acromion. The tip of the needle should be directed toward the contralateral nipple (**Fig. 3**). The steroid mixture should flow freely into the space.[30] Lack of free flow may indicate an impacted needle tip, and the needle should be withdrawn slightly.

ELBOW

The elbow joint comprises the articulations of the humerus, the radius, and the ulna. There is 1 commonly used approach to aspiration and injection of the joint, and success depends on proper landmark identification. For this procedure the patient may be placed in a semirecumbent position with the elbow flexed at 45°.

The lateral epicondyle of the humerus, the lateral aspect of the olecranon, and the head of the radius describe a triangle, the center of which allows percutaneous access to the elbow joint. The needle is inserted and directed toward the medial epicondyle[31]

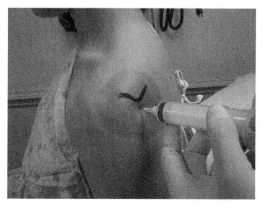

Fig. 2. Posterior approach to the shoulder. Line identifies the posterior and lateral aspects of the acromion.

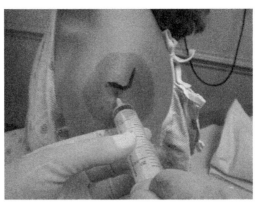

Fig. 3. Injection into the subacromial space. Line indicates posterior and lateral aspect of acromion. Note direction of needle.

(**Fig. 4**). If bony resistance is encountered, the needle should be pulled back slightly and redirected. After aspiration, mixture should flow easily into the joint space.

TECHNIQUE

If additional syringes are needed during aspiration or if therapeutic injection is to be performed, the intraarticular needle may be secured and held steady by application of a sterile hemostat or other device. This procedure allows changeover of the syringes while maintaining needle positioning and minimizing excess movement within the joint space.

On withdrawal of the needle the area should be dressed. Joints with large effusions may benefit from pressure dressings to decrease reaccumulation of fluid. Relative rest of the involved joint for 24 to 48 hours after the procedure is commonly recommended. The procedure, the anticipated course, and plans for follow-up should be discussed with the patient.

Occasionally, after use of intraarticular anesthetic, the patient may experience an episode of rebound pain several hours after the procedure. This pain can occur as the initial anesthetic effect wears off, and can be distressing for the patient. Reviewing this possibility may spare the patient and physician a concerned late-night phone call.

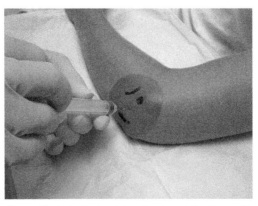

Fig. 4. Injection of elbow. Circle indicates lateral epicondyle. Upper line is the radial head and lower line is lateral border of olecranon.

SUMMARY

Athrocentesis and therapeutic joint injection is a safe, useful, and perhaps underused primary care procedure. Fluid collection and analysis from a joint with an effusion of unclear cause is an important part of appropriate management. Treatment with therapeutic joint injection can give patients significant, rapid, localized pain relief.

REFERENCES

1. Punzi L, Cimmino M, Frizziero L, et al. Italian Society of Rheumatology (SIR) recommendations for performing arthrocentesis. Reumatismo 2007;59(3): 227–34.
2. Punzi L, Oliviero F. Arthrocentesis and synovial fluid analysis in clinical practice. Ann N Y Acad Sci 2009;1154:152–8.
3. Wise C. Arthrocentesis and injection of joints and soft tissues. In: Harris ED, Bud RC, Genovese MC, et al, editors, Kelley's textbook of rheumatology, vol. 1. Philadelphia: WB Saunders; 2005. p. 692–709.
4. Thumboo J, O'Duffy JD. A prospective study of the safety of joint injection and soft tissue aspirations and injections in patients taking warfarin sodium. Arthritis Rheum 1998;41:736–9.
5. Glaser D, Schildhorn J, Bartolozzi A, et al. Do you really know what is on the tip of your needle? The inadvertent introduction of skin into a joint [abstract]. Arthritis Rheum 2000;43:S149.
6. Swan A, Amer H, Dieppe P. The value of synovial fluid assays in the diagnosis of joint disease: a literature survey. Ann Rheum Dis 2002;61:493–8.
7. McGillicuddy D, Shah K, Friedberg R, et al. How sensitive is the synovial fluid white blood cell count in diagnosing septic arthritis? Am J Emerg Med 2007; 25(7):749–52.
8. Margaretten M, Kohlwes J, Moore D, et al. Does this adult patient have septic arthritis? JAMA 2007;297:1478–88.
9. Cooper C, Cawley MID. Bacterial arthritis in an English Health District; a 10-year review. Ann Rheum Dis 1986;45:458–63.
10. Shmerling R. Synovila fluid analysis. A critical reappraisal. Rheum Dis Clin North Am 1994;20:503.
11. Ho G Jr. Infectious disorders. In: Klippel JH, editor. Primer on the rheumatic diseases. 13th edition. New York: Springer Science; 2008. p. 271–6.
12. Garcia-De LaTorre I. Gonococcal and non gonococcal arthritis. Rheum Dis Clin North Am 2009;35:63–73.
13. Shah K, Spear J, Nathanson LA, et al. Does the presence of crystal arthritis rule out septic arthritis? J Emerg Med 2007;32(1):23–6.
14. Weitoft T, Uddenfeldt P. Importance of synovial fluid aspiration when injecting intra-articular corticosteroids. Ann Rheum Dis 2000;59:233–5.
15. Furtado R, Olivera L, Natour J. Polyarticular corticosteroid injection versus systemic administration in treatment of rheumatoid arthritis patients: a randomized controlled study. J Rheumatol 2005;32:1691–8.
16. Hetland M, Stengaard-Petersen K, Junker P, et al. Combination treatment with methotrexate, cyclosporine, and intraarticular betamethasone compared with methotrexate and intraarticular betamethasone in early active rheumatoid arthritis: an investigator-initiated, multicenter, randomized, double-blind, parallel-group, placebo controlled study. Arthritis Rheum 2006;54:1401–9.
17. Stephens M, Beutler A, O'Connor F. Musculoskeletal injections: a review of the evidence. Am Fam Physician 2008;78(8):971–6.

18. Bannuru R, Natov N, Obadan I, et al. Therapeutic trajectory of hyaluronic acid versus corticosteroids in the treatment of knee osteoarthritis: a systematic review and meta-analysis. Arthritis Care Res 2009;61(12):1704–11.
19. Centeno LM, Moore ME. Preferred intraarticular corticosteroid and associated practice: a survey of members of the American College of Rheumatology. Arthritis Care Res 1994;7(3):151–5.
20. Ostensson A, Geborek P. Septic arthritis as a non-surgical complication in rheumatoid arthritis: relation to disease severity and therapy. Br J Rheumatol 1991;30:35–8.
21. Wittich C, Ficalora R, Mason T, et al. Musculoskeletal injection. Mayo Clin Proc 2009;84(9):831–7.
22. Zuber T. Knee joint aspiration and injection. Am Fam Physician 2002;66(8): 1497–501.
23. Cardone DA, Tallia AF. Joint and soft tissue injection. Am Fam Physician 2002; 66(2):283–9.
24. Habib G. The systemic effects of intra-articular corticosteroid. Clin Rheumatol 2009;28(7):749–56.
25. Lazarevic MB, Skosey JL, Djordjevic-Denic G, et al. Reduction of cortisol levels after single intra-articular and intramuscular steroid injection. Am J Med 1995; 99(370):373.
26. Lo IK, Sciore P, Chung M, et al. Local anesthetics induce chondrocyte death in bovine articular cartilage disks in a dose- and duration-dependent manner. Arthroscopy 2009;25(7):707–15.
27. Takeno K, Kobayashi S, Miyazaki T, et al. Lidocaine cytotoxicity to the zygapophysial joints in rabbits: changes in cell viability and proteoglycan metabolism in vitro. Spine 2009;34(26):e945–51.
28. Uziel Y, Berkovitch M, Gazarian M, et al. Evaluation of eutectic lidocaine/prilo-caine cream (EMLA) for steroid joint injection in children with juvenile rheumatoid arthritis; a double-blind, randomized, placebo controlled trial. J Rheumatol 2003; 30:594.
29. Sibbett W, Peisacovich V, Michael A, et al. Does sonographic needle guidance affect the clinical outcome of intraarticular injections? J Rheumatol 2009;36(9): 1892–902.
30. Tallia AF, Cardone DA. Diagnostic and therapeutic injection of the shoulder region. Am Fam Physician 2003;67(6):1271–8.
31. Cardone DA, Tallia AF. Diagnostic and therapeutic injection of the elbow region. Am Fam Physician 2002;66(11):2097–101.
32. Matthews CJ, Coakley G. Septic arthritis: current diagnostic and therapeutic algorithm. Curr Opin Rheumatol 2008;20:457.
33. Ross JJ. Septic Arthritis. Infect Dis Clin North Am 2005;19:799–817.
34. Frazee BW, Fee C, Lambert L. How common is MRSA in adult septic arthritis? Ann Emerg Med 2009;54(5):695–700.
35. Hall S, Buchbinder R. Do imaging methods that guide needle placement improve outcome? Ann Rheum Dis 2004;63(9):1007–8.
36. Stephens MB, Beutler AI, O'Connor FG. Musculoskeletal Injections: a review of the evidence. Am Fam Physician 2008;40(8):539.
37. Rosen P, Chan T, Vilke GM, et al. Atlas of Emergency Procedures. Philadelphia: Mosby Inc; 2001. p. 232–40.
38. Tintinalli JE, Gabor KD, Stapczynski JS. Emergency Medicine. 5th edition. New York: McGraw-Hill; 2000. p. 913.

Crystal Arthropathies: Recognizing and Treating "The Gouch"

David M. Quillen, MD

KEYWORDS

- Gout • Uric acid • Allopurinol • Febuxostat
- Management • Colchicine

Gout is collective name for disorders caused by the formation and deposition of monosodium urate crystals (uric acid). Patients frequently describe the joint pain caused by the uric acid crystals as "the gouch." Gout has been a disease described in history as the disease of kings. Famous people who have suffered from gout include Alexander the Great, Charlemagne, Henry VIII, Benjamin Franklin, Alexander Hamilton, Voltaire, Isaac Newton, and Charles Darwin.[1] It is twice as common among men as women and is the most common cause of inflammatory arthritis in men. An unfortunate perception is that gout is a self-induced disease from dietary excess. Although there is dietary influence on gout and gout flairs, the disease has a genetic basis and its cause is much more complex than simply consuming in excess.

PATHOPHYSIOLOGY

Uric acid is the end product of purine metabolism and is predominantly excreted in urine and, to a lesser extent, in the gastrointestinal (GI) tract (<30%). There are many physiologic factors that affect uric acid excretion, including genetics, drugs, hormones, renal function, and concomitant diseases. In most mammals, the enzyme urate oxidase breaks uric acid down into allantoin (more soluble and easily excreted). Humans lost the ability to produce urate oxidase during primate evolution. The humanoid urate oxidase gene was inactivated by 2 separate mutations, one in the promoter region and the second in the coding region.[2]

Hyperuricemia is necessary for gout to develop (>6.8 mg/dL). The higher the level and the longer it is increased, the more likely acute and chronic gout will develop. Genetics plays a significant role in the development of gout. The 3 main factors for increased urate levels are overproduction, underexcretion, and possibly increased intake. When uric acid levels are high enough needle-shaped monosodium urate crystals form. The crystals commonly deposit in tissues with limited blood flow, such as

Department of Community Health and Family Medicine, University of Florida, 625 SW 4th Avenue, Gainesville, FL 32601, USA
E-mail address: quillen@ufl.edu

Prim Care Clin Office Pract 37 (2010) 703–711
doi:10.1016/j.pop.2010.07.008
0095-4543/10/$ – see front matter © 2010 Elsevier Inc. All rights reserved.

tendons, cartilage, ligaments, bursa, and the skin in areas that are cooler or around distal joints. Tophi are large deposits that usually develop in the skin. In severe chronic hyperuricemia, crystals can develop in large joints and in the kidneys, causing renal stones.

EPIDEMIOLOGY

Estimates of how many people suffer from gout vary with different studies.[3] However, the prevalence seems to have increased and has possibly doubled in the past 3 decades. Based on self-reporting (probably an overestimation), 6.1 million Americans currently suffer from gout (1%–2% of the adult population[4]). Gout is more common in men, particularly at younger ages (35–55 years). As women go through menopause, the incidence steadily increases, and it almost equals the rate in men by age 75 years.

Examination of 2 large observational studies (Health Professions Follow Up Study [HPFS] and the National Health and Nutrition Examination Survey III [NHANES III]) showed that different dietary patterns do affect gout rates[5] (evidence level B). Diets high in meat, fish, beer, and high-fructose soft drinks are linked with a higher incidence of gout in middle-aged men. Diets high in coffee, vitamin C, and possibly low-fat dairy products were linked with reduced rates in the same population. Previously suspected foods (other proteins, wine, and purine-rich vegetables) were found to have little effect.[6]

Despite the effect of diet, the primary problem for patients is uric acid metabolism and excretion, and hyperuricemia. Ten percent of patients make too much because of an error in purine metabolism (overproducers). In the other 90% of gout sufferers, hyperuricemia comes from insufficient uric acid excretion (underexcretors). There are many causes for underexcretion of uric acid, including genetics, dietary intake, renal function, and medications (diuretics, low-dose aspirin, and niacin). The striking increase in gout with age can be attributed to comorbid and contributing conditions such as cardiovascular disease, hypertension, and chronic renal dysfunction.

CLINICAL PRESENTATION

Gout has 4 fundamental stages[7]: asymptomatic hyperuricemia (stage 1), periodic acute gout flairs (stage 2) with asymptomatic susceptible periods (stage 3 or the inter-critical period), and chronic gout with or without tophi (stage 4). Tophi are nodular masses of urate crystals deposited in various soft tissues of the body. Classically, tophi develop over the first metatarsophalangeal joint, but can occur almost anywhere in the body. Hyperuricemia must be present for gout to develop. A uric acid level of more than 6.8 mg/dL is the physiologic point at which uric acid saturation occurs and the development of crystals begins. However, not all patients with hyperuricemia develop gout. In an analysis of data from The Veterans Administrative Normative Aging Study,[8] investigators found that, as the uric acid level increased, so did the incident of gout. The annual incidence of gout was found to be 4.9% for patients with uric acid levels more than 9 mg/dL, compared with 0.5% for uric acid levels of 7 to 8 mg/dL and 0.1% for patients with uric acid levels less than 7 mg/dL. The cumulative 5-year risk for patients with uric acid levels more than 9 mg/dL was 22%. Based just on increased uric acid levels, routine treatment of asymptomatic increase was not considered to be warranted. Age, hypertension, body mass index, cholesterol level, and alcohol intake were also found to be strong predictors of gout development. Patients with hypertension had a 3 times higher incidence of gout for the same uric acid levels. Hyperuricemia, gout, and the metabolic syndrome are connected[9]; however, it is unclear whether hyperuricemia alone contributes to the development of hypertension, diabetes, and cardiovascular disease or is a consequence of these diseases. It is hoped that future research will help resolve the confusion and provide recommendations to treat asymptomatic hyperuricemia to help prevent hypertension, renal dysfunction, and atherosclerotic disease.

Acute gouty arthritis (stage 2) usually first develops in a single joint (monoarticular arthritis, 90%) with the first metatarsophalangeal joint being the most common. Uric acid levels must be high enough that crystals have formed around joints and then are release into the joint. Minor trauma is a known trigger for acute gout attacks. Medical stress, including pneumonia, other infections, strokes, myocardial infarction, and surgery have also been implicated. Thiazide diuretics can increase uric acid levels and rapid lowering of uric acid (urate-lowering therapy) can trigger an acute flare. However, many attacks have no obvious trigger.

Gout can present both typically and atypically. In a typical presentation, the pain is severe, accompanied by swelling and tenderness that reaches a maximum in 6 to 12 hours. The pain may be so severe that patients are unwilling to bear weight on the affected limb. The classic description is that the weight of the bed sheet is too painful to bear. Patients may also experience systemic effects including fever and malaise. Initial untreated attacks usually resolve in 3 to 14 days, and untreated repeat attacks can last much longer. The rates of recurrent attacks are highly variable. Sixty percent of patients have a repeat flair in the first year, 78% within 2 years, and 84% in 3 years.[7] Less than 10% of patients do not have a recurrence in a 10-year period. Gout flairs occur more frequently in lower-extremity joints, but have been described in all joints. In time, and with repeated flairs, other joints become involved and multiarticular flairs can occur.

In chronic or advance gout (stage 4), the deposition of crystals continues. Patients can develop destruction of joints, development of tophi, and persistent and chronic flairs. Why patients progress at different rates, and how quickly they progress from asymptomatic hyperuricemia to acute flairs and then to chronic gout, remain unclear.

DIAGNOSIS AND DIFFERENTIAL

Acute monoarticular arthritis is a common clinical presentation.[10] The most common diagnosis is an acute gout flair, septic arthritis, and acute rheumatoid arthritis. Other diagnoses can present with similar presentations and include osteoarthritis, pseudogout, reactive arthritis (Reiter syndrome), lupus, psoriatic arthritis, adjacent soft tissue infection or cellulitis, spontaneous hemoarthrosis, tuberculosis, aseptic necrosis, synovial chondromatosis, and unknown causes.[10] Definitive diagnosis of gout can only be made by examining synovial fluid and identifying bright, negatively birefringent needlelike crystals that are intracellular and extracellular under polarizing microscopy. A clinical diagnosis of gout is probably adequate in patients who have recurrent typical presentations and increased uric acid levels.[11] For patients with a first-time flair, reasonable attempts to obtain synovial fluid should be pursued. Missing the diagnosis of a septic joint can have significant consequences.

TREATMENT: ACUTE FLAIRS

The goal of treatment is to minimize or eliminate the acute flairs, prevent joint destruction, and minimize side effects. For acute flairs, quick symptomatic treatment is important. For recurrent flairs, prevention becomes the goal. For patient with chronic tophi, reabsorption and resolution of the tophi is the goal.

Three different medication classes are commonly used for treating acute flairs: nonsteroidal antiinflammatory drugs (NSAIDs), colchicine, and steroids. NSAIDs are frequently used and have a quick onset of action. Safety issues are of concern, particularly in patients who have renal dysfunction or a potential for GI bleeding. Indomethicin has been the most commonly used, but many other short–half-life NSAIDs are equally effective. cyclooxygenase-2 (COX II) inhibitors are equally effective, and may have an improved safety profile[12] (etoricoxib is only available in Europe; level of evidence B2, single randomized controlled trial of good quality).

The medicinal value of the plant containing colchicine has been recognized for more than 2000 years. Colchicine is a toxic alkaloid extracted from the plant *Colchicum autumnale* (commonly known as autumn crocus, meadow saffron, or naked lady) and was first isolated in 1820 by 2 French chemists, PS Pelletier and J Caventon. Colchicine can be used during acute flairs and chronic suppression. Colchicine inhibits white cell migration and activation and is effective for acute flairs and chronic prophylaxis. Colchicine has been available in many generic forms and used for many years without United States Food and Drug Administration (FDA) approval for the treatment of gout. The FDA ordered the discontinuation of intravenous (IV) colchicine products in February 2008 in response to safety concerns. In 2006, the FDA started an initiative to bring unapproved products such as colchicine under its regulatory framework, with a goal of assuring that all marketed drugs meet modern standards for safety, effectiveness, quality, and labeling. URL Pharma commissioned several studies that demonstrated the safety and efficacy of colchicine in gout. The FDA-approved Colcrys (a brand name for colchicine) in July 2009 and gave URL Pharma an exclusive 3-year marketing right for treating acute gout flairs and a 7-year exclusive right for familial Mediterranean fever. Colchicine for chronic gout prophylaxis was not included in the FDA action. As a consequence of FDA approval and numerous lawsuits initiated by URL Pharma, the only colchicine readily available is Colcrys at $5 per dose (up from the generic cost of pennies per tablet).[13]

For acute flairs, the FDA-approved dose of colchicine is 1.2 mg (2 tablets) followed by a third tablet 1 hour later. Colchicine can be use for prophylaxis and is dosed at 0.6 mg daily or twice a day (not FDA approved, but general consensus). The major side effect is GI, with nausea and diarrhea. Dosing colchicine 0.6 mg every hour until pain resolves or GI side effects develop should no longer be recommended. Significant drug interactions can occur with other medications that inhibit the CYP3A4 and/or P-glycoprotein (P-gp) with increased risk of colchicine toxicity. Patients with renal dysfunction should also have the dose reduced (limited to 0.3 mg/d for severe renal dysfunction or dialysis) and used with caution.

Corticosteroids can also be used for the treatment of acute gout flairs. Oral steroids compare well with NSAIDs in acute flairs.[14] Using oral steroids for 5 days (30–55 mg of prednisolone or its equivalent) is an option for patients with renal disease or intolerance to either NSAIDs or colchicine. Intra-articular corticosteroid is also an effective way of managing an acute flair. Not all joints are accessible for injection, but for those that are, not only does it provide an opportunity for fluid analysis, but injecting (10–40 mg for a knee) triamcinalone mixed with lidocaine offers immediate pain relief and treatment of the flair. The use of synthetic adenocorticotropic hormone (ACTH) has been described.[15] However, there are no clear dosing regimens, and the expense and availability of synthetic ACTH (corticotropin) limit its use.

TREATMENT: CHRONIC GOUT

The long-term clinical goal of chronic gout management is to minimize or eliminate recurrent flairs, reabsorb any tophi, and prevent joint destruction (**Table 1**). Reducing uric acid levels to less than 6 mg/dL reduces or eliminates most gout flairs and slowly

Table 1
Treatment options

Acute Gout Flair	Average Dose	Concerns
NSAIDs	Indomethicin 50 mg three times a day Naproxen 500 mg twice a day Ibuprofen 800 mg three times a day Many others available	Age, history of GI bleed, renal dysfunction
COX II	Celecoxib 200 mg twice a day[27]	Same concerns as the NSAIDs, fewer GI side effects, potential cardiac toxicity
Colchicine	1.2 mg at onset of flair, titrate down	Lower dose effective with fewer GI side effects
Steroid, oral	Prednisolone 35–55 mg per day or equivalent	Chronic use of steroids should be avoided
Steroid, injection	Triamcinalone 10–40 mg intra-articular or equivalent	Could complicate a septic joint, practitioners need to be comfortable that they can access the joint
ACTH	40 IU intramuscular/IV/ subcutaneous No clear dosing regime	Given other options and availability, not a recommended option
Chronic Gout		
Colchicine	0.6 mg per day	
Allopurinol	Initial dose 100–300 mg by mouth per day, can titrate up to 800 mg/day	Dose adjustment for renal insufficiency and titrate to get uric acid level less than 6 mg/dL. Significant toxicity
Probenecid	250 mg twice a day first week, then 500 mg twice a day Titrate to max of 1000 mg twice a day	Avoid in patients with chronic kidney disease or a history of renal stones. 24-hour urine required before initiation
Febuxostat	40 mg/d and can increase to 80 mg/day	Recommended for patients with intolerance to allopurinol
Rasburicase (urate oxidase)	0.2 mg/kg/dose IV	Reserved for specialty services for the most refractory cases

resolves most tophi. Lifestyle modifications (exercise, dietary modification, and reduction in alcohol consumption) have been found to reduce the uric acid level at best by 15%,[6] which would mean that most patients would still need medications to prevent recurrent flairs and achieve a uric acid level of less than 6 mg/dL. However, no significant clinical trials have demonstrated lifestyle modification as an effective treatment of gout. It is still prudent for physicians to recommend lifestyle modifications to their patients. The benefits are clear in associated metabolic diseases (diabetes mellitus, hypertension, and so forth) and it may reduce the amount of medication needed to control gout.

Patients should be started on uric acid–lowering medication if they have 2 or more gout flairs in a year, have any of the advanced signs of gout,[4] and are diagnosed as overproducers (90% of gout sufferers are undersecretors). These advanced signs include tophi, the combination of gout and urolithiasis, gout that is severe or difficult to treat, or if gout is found in combination with stage 3 chronic kidney disease, congestive heart failure, or persistent gouty arthritis. Starting uric acid–lowering therapies during an acute flair often makes it worse and can increase the number of gouty attacks during the first 6 months of therapy. Destabilization of the synovial crystals and remodeling is a generally accepted, but unproven, theory for why uric acid–lowering treatment temporarily increases flairs. Some have recommended using prophylactic NSAIDs or colchicine for the first 6 months of therapy.[4,16] There are obvious risks with 6 months of continuous NSAID therapy. With the limited availability of low-cost colchicine, and alternative to prophylaxis would be to provide NSAIDs, colchicine, or short-course oral steroids for patients to have at home and take when a flair occurs.

Probenecid and benzbromarone are effective uricosuric medications that inhibit urate anion reabsorption by the proximal renal tubules and effectively increase the urinary excretion of uric acid. Benzbromarone is not available in the United States because of concerns about hepatotoxicity. Probenecid and benzbromarone medications are effective and well tolerated in patients with normal renal function and no history of kidney stones. Uricosuric medications are not appropriate for patients who overproduce uric acid. Patients should have a 24-hour urine and show less than 800 mg of uric while on a normal purine diet[17] before being started. Because probenecid can cause nephrolithiasis, patients should maintain adequate urine output and should avoid doses of aspirin greater than 81 mg because of concerns about decreasing the efficacy.

The starting dose for probenecid is 250 mg twice a day for the first week, increasing to 500 mg twice a day starting the second week. The goal for treatment is to obtain a uric acid level less than 6 mg/dL. If that level is not achieved, the dose can be titrated up to 1000 mg twice a day. If a serum uric acid level of 6 mg/dL is still not achieved after reaching the maximum dose, the addition of allopurinol or febuxostat can help. Probenecid is probably underused because of the need for the 24-hour urine before initiating treatment. Complications include the development of kidney stones and a rare, but serious, anaphylactic reaction. Consistent with all uric acid–lowering therapy, probenecid can increase the number of gouty flairs during the first 6 months of therapy.

Allopurinol has been used effectively for more than 40 years. It is a purine analogue that blocks the xanthine oxidase enzyme that converts xanthine to uric acid. Xanthine is easily excreted in the urine. Allopurinol has been the medication of choice for most chronic gout sufferers. It works effectively for either underexcretors or overproducers and can be started without 24-hour urine testing.

The major concern and risk for patients is the development of allopurinol hypersensitivity syndrome (AHS). AHS is uncommon, with an incidence between 0.1% and 0.4%, although it is common enough to be of concern. AHS can be limited to a severe skin reaction similar to Steven-Johnson syndrome or can include systemic or multiorgan involvement. Mortality can be up to 25% in patients who develop AHS. Confirmed risk factors for AHS include allopurinol started within a few months, chronic kidney disease, and HLA-B58 allele in patients with Han Chinese and European ancestry. Possible risk factors also include use of thiazide diuretics, high dose in comparison to renal function, and patients with increased uric acid without gout.[18] Other side effects can include a rash with puritis in about 2% (up to 20% if combined with amoxicillin or ampicillin), occasionally bone marrow suppression, mild increase of liver enzymes (direct hepatotoxicity is rare), and GI side effects (diarrhea and nausea). Patients who develop a rash but are not concurrently taking amoxicillin or ampicillin should stop taking allopurinol immediately. Patients who become sensitized to allopurinol can be considered for desensitization regimes under careful monitoring by a clinician experienced in the process, risks, and benefits. With the release of febuxostat, desensitization regimes may no longer be necessary except in the most refractory patients or those who have reacted to both medications.

Dosing guidelines for allopurinol vary.[18,19] Older guidelines are conservative with concerns for the development of AHS in patients with renal insufficiency and when titrating to higher doses in patients with normal renal function. Only 40% of patients with normal renal function given the standard allopurinol 300 mg/day achieve good control or uric acid levels less than 6 mg/dL. The older guidelines limited the ability to titrate the allopurinol dose to achieve an adequate reduction in serum uric acid.[18] When the earlier recommendations were critically reviewed, investigators considered it was safe to make recommendations that are less conservative and more flexible in titrating the dose of allopurinol.[4] Research and expert opinion now supports a treat-to-target strategy.[20]

The starting dose for patients with normal renal function is 100 mg/day. The dose should be increased weekly until the uric acid at less than 6 mg/dL. Maximum dose is 800 mg/day. When prescribing more than 300 mg/day, divided dosing decreases GI side effects. The starting dose for patients with renal dysfunction is also 100 mg/day. Titration should occur at a slower and more conservative pace, with increases of 50 mg rather than 100 mg. The maximum dose for patients with creatinine clearance of less than 60 mL/min should in most cases be 300 mg/day or less. Titration schedule and uric acid–lowering strategy should be individualized for each patient with chronic renal dysfunction.

Febuxostat was approved by the FDA in February 2009 for chronic treatment of gout. Touted as the first new treatment of gout in more than 40 years, febuxostat is the second xanthine oxidase inhibitor available. Febuxostat is chemically different from allopurinol, and does not have a purine core structure. In the past 5 years, numerous clinical trials have been conducted comparing feboxostat with allopurinol and with placebo.[21–26] Febuxostat compares well with standard allopurinol 300 mg/day dosing. It shows efficacy in patients with renal dysfunction and has good long-term gout control with a tolerable side effect profile. It is primarily metabolized in the liver by oxidation and glucuronidation. No dosing adjustment is needed for renal dysfunction or for hepatic dysfunction. Caution is recommended for patients with CrCl less than 30 mL/min and it has not been studied in patients on hemodialysis. Numerous side effects have been reported, including rash, diarrhea, and increased liver enzymes. Unlike allopurinol, no severe skin reactions were reported. The starting dose of feboxostat is 40 mg/day. It can be titrated up to 80 mg/day and is approved by the FDA for the 40 mg and 80 mg dose. In Europe, it has been approved up to the 120 mg/day dose. Current recommendations are that feboxostat be used in patients who are intolerant of allopurinol, which makes sense from a financial perspective. Current Internet prices for febuxostat are around $5.00 for a 40 mg tablet, and allopurinol 300 mg is around 20 cents.

Rasburicase is a recombinant urate oxidase that has been approved by the FDA for initial prevention of tumor lysis syndrome in pediatric and adult patients with leukemia, lymphoma, and solid tumor malignancies.[2,7] It has been used experimentally with patients who have severe tophaceous gout refractory to allopurinol and who have end stage renal disease, and renal transplant and heart transplant recipients. Rasburicase has been shown to be effective in debulking large tophi and bringing previously refractory cases under control. There are significant safety concerns and side effects with injected biologic agents such as rasburicase, and such treatments should be reserved for only the most refractory cases, and then only under specialty services.

Table 2
Key elements in treating gout

	Key Elements	Level of Evidence
1	Make the diagnosis (bright, negatively birefringent needlelike crystals from joint aspiration)	C3
2	Treat the acute flair: colchicine, NSAIDs or oral steroids	C3
3	If a patient has 2 or more flairs in a year, treat for chronic gout	C3
4	Lifestyle modifications may help	C3
5	Do not start uric acid–lowering medication during an acute flair	A1
6	Treat to target, titrate, and get the uric acid level less than 6 mg/mL	C3
7	Expect an increase in flairs during the first 6 mo of uric acid–lowering therapy. Prescribe prophylaxis or prescribe flair treatment to have on hand	A2, C3
8	Recognize the serious side effect potential of allopurinol	
9	Probenecid is an effective and well-tolerated medication for patients with normal renal function. A 24-h urine is needed to show undersecretion	C3
10	Febuxostat is an option for patients intolerant to allopurinol	A1

SUMMARY

Gout is a common disease and the prevalence is increasing. Chronic hyperuricemia (uric acid serum levels of more than 6.8 mg/dL) is a key feature. Treating to a target uric acid level of 6.0 mg/dL is recommended. In addition to cochicine, probenecid, and allopurinol, feboxostat is a new option for urate-lowering therapy. **Table 2** shows a summary of the key elements clinicians that need to treat in this prevalent disease.

REFERENCES

1. Gower T. Like Charlemagne, you've got gout. New York: The New York Times; 2005.
2. Vogt B. Urate oxidase (rasburicase) for treatment of severe tophaceous gout. Nephrol Dial Transplant 2005;20(2):431–3.
3. Lawrence RC, Felson DT, Helmick CG, et al. Estimates of the prevalence of arthritis and other rheumatic conditions in the United States. Part II. Arthritis Rheum 2008;58(1):26–35.
4. Terkeltaub R. Update on gout: new therapeutic strategies and options. Nat Rev Rheumatol 2010;6:30–8.
5. Hak AE, Choi HK. Lifestyle and gout. Curr Opin Rheumatol 2008;20(2):179–86.
6. Lee SJ, Terkeltaub RA, Kavanaugh A. Recent developments in diet and gout. Curr Opin Rheumatol 2006;18(2):193–8.
7. Mandell BF. Clinical manifestations of hyperuricemia and gout [review]. Cleve Clin J Med 2008;75(Suppl 5):S5–8.
8. Campion EW, Glynn RJ, DeLabry LO. Asymptomatic hyperuricemia. Risks and consequences in the Normative Aging Study. Am J Med 1987;82(3):421–6.
9. Feig DI, Kang DH, Johnson RJ. Uric acid and cardiovascular risk. N Engl J Med 2008;359(17):1811–21.

10. Ma L, Cranney A, Holroyd-Leduc JM. Acute monoarthritis: what is the cause of my patient's painful swollen joint? CMAJ 2009;180(1):59–65.

11. Zhang W, Doherty M, Pascual E, et al. EULAR evidence based recommendations for gout. Part I: diagnosis. Report of a task force of the Standing Committee for International Clinical Studies Including Therapeutics (ESCISIT). Ann Rheum Dis 2006;65(10):1301–11.

12. Rubin BR, Burton R, Navarra S, et al. Efficacy and safety profile of treatment with etoricoxib 120 mg once daily compared with indomethacin 50 mg three times daily in acute gout: a randomized controlled trial. Arthritis Rheum 2004;50(2):598–606.

13. Rockoff JD. An old gout drug gets a new life and a new price, riling patients. Wall St J 2010. Available at: online.wsj.com. Accessed April 12, 2010.

14. Janssens HJ, Janssen M, van de Lisdonk EH, et al. Use of oral prednisolone or naproxen for the treatment of gout arthritis: a double-blind, randomised equivalence trial. Lancet 2008;371(9627):1854–60.

15. Schlesinger N. Overview of the management of acute gout and the role of adrenocorticotropic hormone. Drugs 2008;68(4):407–15.

16. Borstad GC, Bryant LR, Abel MP, et al. Colchicine for prophylaxis of acute flares when initiating allopurinol for chronic gouty arthritis. J Rheumatol 2004;31(12):2429–32.

17. Keith MP, Gilliland WR. Updates in the management of gout. Am J Med 2007; 120(3):221–4.

18. Chao J, Terkeltaub R. A critical reappraisal of allopurinol dosing, safety, and efficacy for hyperuricemia in gout. Curr Rheumatol Rep 2009;11(2):135–40.

19. Hande KR, Noone RM, Stone WJ. Severe allopurinol toxicity. Description and guidelines for prevention in patients with renal insufficiency. Am J Med 1984; 76(1):47–56.

20. Reinders MK, Haagsma C, Jansen TL, et al. A randomised controlled trial on the efficacy and tolerability with dose escalation of allopurinol 300–600 mg/day versus benzbromarone 100–200 mg/day in patients with gout. Ann Rheum Dis 2009;68(6):892–7.

21. Becker MA, Schumacher HR Jr, Wortmann RL, et al. Febuxostat, a novel nonpurine selective inhibitor of xanthine oxidase: a twenty-eight-day, multicenter, phase II, randomized, double-blind, placebo-controlled, dose-response clinical trial examining safety and efficacy in patients with gout. Arthritis Rheum 2005; 52(3):916–23.

22. Becker MA, Schumacher HR Jr, Wortmann RL, et al. Febuxostat compared with allopurinol in patients with hyperuricemia and gout. Engl J Med 2005;353(23): 2450–61.

23. Schumacher HR Jr, Becker MA, Wortmann RL, et al. Effects of febuxostat versus allopurinol and placebo in reducing serum urate in subjects with hyperuricemia and gout: a 28-week, phase III, randomized, double-blind, parallel-group trial. Arthritis Rheum 2008;59(11):1540–8.

24. Schumacher HR Jr, Becker MA, Lloyd E, et al. Febuxostat in the treatment of gout: 5-yr findings of the FOCUS efficacy and safety study. Rheumatology (Oxford) 2009;48(2):188–94.

25. Becker MA, Schumacher HR, MacDonald PA, et al. Clinical efficacy and safety of successful longterm urate lowering with febuxostat or allopurinol in subjects with gout. J Rheumatol 2009;36(6):1273–82.

26. Becker MA, Schumacher HR, Espinoza LR, et al. The urate-lowering efficacy and safety of febuxostat in the treatment of the hyperuricemia of gout: the CONFIRMS trial. Arthritis Res Ther 2010;12(2):R63.

27. Cochrane DJ, Jarvis B, Keating GM. Etoricoxib. Drugs 2002;62(18):2637–51.

Beyond Osteoarthritis: Recognizing and Treating Infectious and Other Inflammatory Arthropathies in Your Practice

Zewdu Haile, MD*, Sanjeeb Khatua, MD

KEYWORDS

• Arthritis • Infection • Primary care • Diagnosis • Management

Key Points	Evidence Rating
About 15% of patients presenting in a primary care clinic have joint pain as their primary complaint.	B
Disseminated gonorrhea is the most common cause of infectious arthritis in sexually active, previously healthy patients.	B
Prompt arthrocentesis, microscopic examination, culture of any purulent material, and appropriate antibiotic therapy are the mainstay of treatment in infectious arthritis.	C
Detailed history, including family history and comprehensive examination, is more useful in accurate diagnosis than expensive laboratory and radiological investigations for noninfectious arthritis.	C
Regarding inflammatory noninfectious arthritis with the potential to cause destructive joint damage, early referral to a subspecialist, when indicated, increases the likelihood of optimal outcome.	C
Nonsteroidal antiinflammatory drugs are the first line of therapeutic agents to reduce pain and swelling in the management of most noninfectious inflammatory arthritis seen in the primary care office.	C

Hinsdale Family Medicine Residency, Hinsdale, IL, USA
* Corresponding author.
E-mail address: Zewdu.Haile.MD@ahss.org

Prim Care Clin Office Pract 37 (2010) 713–727
doi:10.1016/j.pop.2010.07.004
0095-4543/10/$ – see front matter

Arthritis (from the Greek word "artron" meaning joint and the Latin word "itis" meaning inflammation) is a disease of the musculoskeletal system, specifically the joints. Arthritis and other rheumatic conditions are the leading causes of disability in the United States.[1] Joint pain is among the most common complaints encountered in family medicine.[2]

Arthritis is a component of more than 100 diseases, the most common form being osteoarthritis. This article concentrates primarily on patients with infectious inflammatory arthritides, which are typically monoarticular, and who are usually seen in the primary care ambulatory setting. Oligoarticular and polyarticular noninfectious inflammatory arthritis (rheumatoid diseases) are discussed briefly later in this article. This discussion is to help differentiate inflammatory from infectious arthritis and to offer recommendations on when to refer patients for expert care. More extensive coverage of these diseases, as well as gout, osteoarthritis, and rheumatoid arthritis (RA), are covered in other articles in this issue.

CLASSIFICATION

Arthritis is characterized by joint pain and inflammation; the latter is characterized by warmth, tenderness, erythema, and swelling or effusion. Arthritis can occur at rest or with activity and may interfere with sleep. Constitutional symptoms are common and may indicate either an infectious or an inflammatory process. Joint pain without inflammation is termed arthralgia and may or may not be prodromal to an arthritic condition. In particular, pain duration of less than 15 minutes is more indicative of arthralgia. Conditions such as sciatica may present with a complaint of joint pain, and a careful examination excludes arthritides as a cause. In addition, diseases such as bacterial endocarditis, which cause disseminated infection, can affect joints as well.

Arthritides are customarily classified as monoarticular, oligoarticular (2 to 4 separate joints), or polyarticular (**Box 1**). Other classifications of the arthritides are symmetric or asymmetric and acute or chronic.

Infectious arthritis is predominantly monoarticular in 80% to 90% of patients[3]; therefore, acute-onset monoarticular involvement should be considered infectious until proved otherwise. A condition that initially seems to be monoarticular may eventually involve multiple joints.

Gout is also a common cause of acute monoarticular arthritis. Sodium urate crystals in the synovium incite the inflammatory response. The metatarsophalangeal joint of the great toe is the classic site, but the midfoot, ankle, knee, wrist, and olecranon bursae are other potential locations. Pseudogout results when crystals of calcium pyrophosphate induce joint inflammation. Pseudogout resembles gout pathologically; however, the attacks are usually less severe. Knees and wrists are the most commonly affected sites.

Immunologically mediated conditions typically cause polyarticular arthritis; however, they may present initially as a monoarticular arthritis. ReA (postinfectious arthritis), ankylosing spondylitis, PsA, and the arthritis of IBD, which are also immunologically mediated conditions, are more likely to present as oligoarticular arthritis.

PATHOGENESIS

Infectious arthritis can result from a bite or trauma, from direct inoculation of bacteria or other organisms during joint surgery, or, rarely, when infection of bone adjacent to the joint extends through the cortex into the joint space. However,

---

Box 1
Classification of arthritis by the number of joints involved and examples

Monoarticular arthritis

    Bacterial arthritis

        Disseminated gonorrheal infection

        Nongonococcal infectious arthritis

        Lyme disease

        Mycobacterial infection

    Viral arthritis

        Human immunodeficiency virus (HIV) infection

        Parvovirus B19 infection

    Gouty arthritis

        Acute gout

        Pseudogout

Oligoarticular arthritis

    Rheumatic fever

    Reactive arthritis (ReA)

    Ankylosing spondylitis

    Psoriatic arthritis (PsA)

    Arthritis associated with inflammatory bowel disease (IBD)

Polyarticular arthritis

    RA

    Systemic lupus erythematosus (SLE)

    Still disease

    Behçet disease

    Sarcoid arthritis (SA)

Data from Ho G Jr. Infectious disorders. In: Klippel JH, Stone JH, Crofford LJ, et al, editors. Primer on the rheumatic diseases. 13th edition. New York: Springer Science; 2008. p. 271–6; and Kaandorp CJE, Kriknen P, Moens HJB, et al. The outcome of bacterial arthritis. A prospective community-based study. Arthritis Rheum 1997;40(5):884–92.

---

in most cases, infectious arthritis arises from hematogenous spread to the joint.[4] Large joints are more commonly affected than small joints, and the hip or the knee is involved in up to 60% of cases.[5] The endotoxins and exotoxins liberated by bacteria and other organisms, the immune complexes formed from the organisms' antigens and host antibodies, and the lysosomal enzymes released by the autolysis of polymorphonuclear (PMN) leucocytes cause considerable damage to the articular synovium.

The process of joint destruction can become irreversible in hours to days; therefore, it is imperative to recognize and manage acute infectious arthritis rapidly while the inflammatory process is still reversible to avoid a chronic disabling outcome of the involved joints, as well as minimize the potential for the development of life-threatening sepsis.

DIAGNOSTIC APPROACH
History and Physical Examination

The patient's history offers important information that must be used to direct further diagnostic investigation (**Table 1**). The presence of constitutional symptoms, which indicate the possibility of sepsis syndrome, should lead to immediate hospitalization and initiation of broad-spectrum antibiotics while pursuing further investigation.[6] All joints are carefully examined to ascertain the location and the extent of the problem. Signs of inflammation are sought (increased warmth, swelling, redness, effusion, all of which are hallmarks of synovitis). Joint-line tenderness, restricted active and passive motion of joints, diminished weight bearing, joint swelling, joint warmth, presence of low- or high-grade fever, and erythema can point to acute infectious arthritis.

Laboratory Investigation

Hematology
Elevated white blood cell (WBC) count with left shift signifies a infectious cause, particularly bacteria.

Table 1
Differentiating between infectious and noninfectious arthritis

	Infectious	Noninfectious
Constitutional Symptoms	High fever Age>60	Consider rheumatoid if constitutional symptoms in addition to low-grade fever Previous urethritis, uveitis suggest ReA
Risk Factors	Skin infections Risky sexual behavior Vaginal or urethral discharge Exposure to gonorrhea Recent intra-articular steroid injection Osteomyelitis	Trauma (consider fracture) Family history of inflammatory arthritis
Numbers and Types of Joints Involved	Single Migratory, consider gonorrhea	Migratory, consider rheumatoid
Characteristics of Pain	Acute Significant local pain	Aggravated by motion and weight bearing (osteoarthritis) Morning stiffness (RA)
Comorbid Conditions	Diabetes mellitus Concurrent RA Immunosuppression Sickle cell disease Chronic renal disease	
Functional Loss or Disability		Chronic and typically not infectious, consider fungi and tuberculosis

Data from Fagan HB. Approach to the patient with acute swollen/painful joint. Clin Fam Pract 2005;7(2):305–19; and Robinson DB, EL-Gabalawy HS. Evaluation of the patient. A. History and physical examination. In: Stone JH, Crofford LJ, editors. Primer on the rheumatic diseases. 13th edition. New York: Springer; 2008. p. 6–14.

Synovial fluid analysis
If synovial fluid is readily obtainable and the diagnosis is uncertain after history taking, physical examination, and standard blood and urine laboratory tests, then synovial fluid analysis should be performed. Arthrocentesis should also be performed in the febrile patient with an acute flare of joint pain who has an already established inflammatory or gouty arthritis and in whom superimposed infectious arthritis is suspected. Contraindications to arthrocentesis include bacteremia, inaccessible joints, joint prosthesis, and overlying infection in soft tissue.

The WBC count, differential WBC count, cultures, gram staining, synovial fluid analysis, and polarized light microscopy to detect gouty crystals are the studies usually performed on synovial fluid.[7,8] Noninflammatory fluids generally have a WBC count of fewer than 2000/μL, with fewer than 75% PMN leukocytes. Negative gram staining and a negative result on culture of synovial fluid do not preclude infectious arthritis. The sensitivities of gram staining and culture are not sufficient to rule out infectious arthritis. Even though synovial fluid leukocytosis shows considerable variation among patients with infectious arthritis, it probably has the best clinical utility in predicting inflammation and therefore infection. In the absence of a definitive diagnosis from gram staining and culture, antibiotic therapy should be initiated if clinical suspicion persists to avoid the serious and life-threatening complications.[4]

Uric acid
Serum uric acid levels are usually elevated in gout. Because asymptomatic hyperuricemia has a high prevalence in the general population, the test has little or no diagnostic value. In addition, normal uric acid levels are fairly common during an attack of gout, especially with polyarticular involvement.

Other tests
If clinical presentation warrants, serologic tests for HIV, hepatitis B and C, Lyme disease, and HLA-B27 can be considered.

Synovial biopsy
In rare instances, the correct diagnosis of the arthritis depends on tissue biopsy results. Indications for synovial biopsy include refractory arthritis, a high degree of suspicion for atypical infectious agents, or evaluation for intra-articular tumors.

Imaging Studies

Plain radiography should be performed when there is suspicion of a potential fracture, osteomyelitis or infiltrative disease from malignancy, or potential deep-seated infections of the spine or hip. If this is the case, it may be prudent to delay arthrocentesis until appropriate imaging techniques can provide an assurance that routine, and not guided, arthrocentesis is indicated. In patients with chronic symptoms, imaging studies are also indicated when localization of the anatomic structure that is causing symptoms is not readily apparent, especially after significant trauma, if there is a loss of joint function (eg, unable to bear weight), if pain continues despite conservative management, if a fracture is suspected, if a deep-seated bone infection of the spine or hip is suspected, or if a history of malignancy is known and infiltrative disease in the joint is suspected. Plain radiographs are not necessary if the clinical presentation is clearly acute RA, SLE, or gout. In suspected infectious arthritis, a serial study may be used to detect characteristic bony changes, such as new subperiosteal bone formation and transcortical sinus tracts. If osteomyelitis is suspected, bone scan or magnetic resonance imaging (MRI) is indicated. A bone scan may be useful when stress fracture or bony metastases are a concern. MRI and computerized tomography (CT) are reserved for patients in whom the diagnosis cannot be made in a less-costly manner, after less-invasive and costly investigations are complete.[9]

Diagnostic Cascade Algorithm

An overview of the diagnostic approach is found in **Fig. 1**.

MANAGEMENT OF INFECTIOUS ARTHRITIS

The positive predictive value for synovial fluid gram staining and culture is less than 50% in gonococcal joint disease. Even in the presence of a negative gram staining results, a recent history of unprotected sex should raise suspicion of this type of

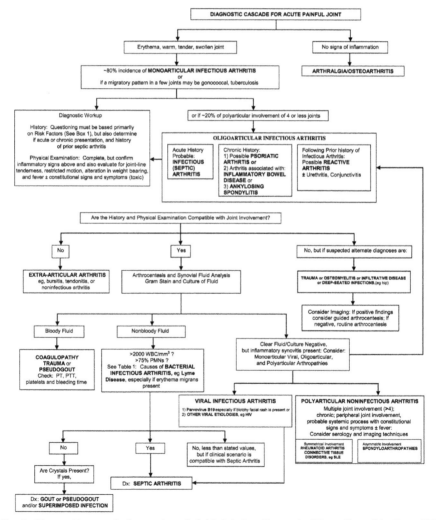

Fig. 1. Diagnostic cascade for acute painful joint. Dx, diagnosis; PT, prothrombin time; PTT, partial thromboplastin time.

arthritis, and simultaneous cultures of the cervix, urethra, and rectum should be obtained. Clinical suspicion of gonococcal arthritis should be heightened if the patient is young (the prevalence is greatest in young women) and the symptoms are polyarticular. In the sexually inactive young person, in the older patient with risk factors as identified in **Table 1**, and in cases of monoarticular symptoms and clinical suspicion of an infectious origin, a more intensive investigation should be undertaken, likely in consultation with an orthopedic specialist. Nongonoccal infectious arthritis has a poor prognosis without joint drainage.

After significant nongonococcal intra-articulate infection has been eliminated as a concern, the patient should be encouraged to rest, immobilize the affected joint, and ice the joint if an effusion is present. If pain is excessive and a diagnosis is not yet established, an analgesic without antiinflammatory effects (acetaminophen or codeine) may be used. Large effusions can recur and may require repeat aspiration. Intra-articular injection of corticosteroids may be indicated after infection is eliminated as a potential cause, especially in traumatic or exercise-induced inflammatory arthritis, some oligoarticular arthropathies,[10] or other unexplained joint effusions.

Acute nongonococcal bacterial arthritis should be managed in consultation with a physician who specializes in the management of such conditions. Therapeutic considerations include the need to wash out the intra-articular space, the need for splinting of the joint, and the need for rehabilitation.[11,12]

Antibiotic Selection in Infectious Arthritis

No randomized controlled studies have evaluated antibiotic regimens for bacterial arthritis before culture results. The initial choice of antimicrobial regimens is based on the coverage of the most likely organism to cause infection in the clinical setting, the gram staining result, and the clinical presentation (**Tables 2** and **3**). Because dosage recommendations change frequently, it is recommended that a reference such as the Sanford Guide to Antibiotic Therapy be consulted before initiating antibiotic therapy. Empiric recommendations have been included in **Table 2** as well.

The length of therapy is based on the results of serial synovial fluid analyses. The presence of sterile fluid and a decreasing total leukocyte count suggest therapeutic improvement. If not, reassessment of the effectiveness of joint drainage and/or an alteration in the antimicrobial regimen should be considered.

Mortality caused by nongonococcal bacterial arthritis depends on the presence of comorbid conditions, such as advanced age, coexistent renal or cardiac disease, and immunosuppression. The mortality rates in most series have ranged from 10% to 15%.[13] Polyarticular infectious arthritis, particularly when caused by *Staphylococcus aureus* infection or in the presence of RA, has an extremely poor prognosis, with mortality rates as high as 50%.[14]

Viral arthritis

Therapy is generally directed at relief of symptoms and maintenance of function. Patients should be treated with analgesic agents (eg, acetaminophen) and nonsteroidal antiinflammatory drugs (NSAIDs) in doses typically used in any inflammatory arthropathy. Physical and occupational therapy may be initiated if required to maintain or improve function. The use of glucocorticoids, orally or by intra-articular injection, should be discouraged because they are of limited utility in this disorder or may mask the disease and the correct diagnosis. Specific antiviral therapy is unnecessary because most viral arthritis are of short duration and self-limited.

Table 2
Gram staining results, potential causative agents, and antibiotic choices

Type of Organism	Specific Pathogen	Antibiotic Choice with Suggested Dosing
Gram-positive cocci	Staphylococcus aureus Staphylococcus epidermis Streptococcus pyogenes Peptostreptococcus	Vancomycin, 30 mg/kg daily in 2 divided doses
Gram-positive bacilli	Listeria monocytogenes Corynebacteria Clostridia	
Gram-negative cocci	Neisseria gonococcus Neisseria meningitides Moraxella	Ceftriaxone, 1 g intravenously once a day until at least 24 h after symptoms and signs resolve, followed by cefixime, 400 mg orally twice daily for 7 d[4] Coexisting genital infection with Chlamydia trachomatis: doxycycline, 100 mg orally twice daily for 7 d, or Zithromax, 1 g orally once a day for 7 d
Gram-negative bacilli	Escherichia coli Pseudomonas aeruginossa Haemophilus influenzae Klebsiella Salmonella Campylobacter Serratia Bacteroides Fusobacteria	Ceftriaxone, 2 g intravenously once daily, or cefotaxime, 2 g intravenously every 8 h For cephalosporin-allergic patients: ciprofloxacin, 400 mg intravenously every 12 h, or 500–750 mg orally twice daily If Pseudomonas suspected: ceftriaxone plus an aminoglycoside pending culture results
Negative gram staining in an immunocompetent patient		Vancomycin, 30 mg/kg daily in 2 divided doses, pending culture results
Negative gram staining in an immunocompromised patient with traumatic, presumed infectious arthritis		Vancomycin plus ceftriaxone pending culture results

Data from Garcia-De LaTorre I. Gonococcal and nongonococcal arthritis. Rheum Dis Clin North Am 2009;35:63–73; and Dubost JJ, Fis I, Denis P, et al. Polyarticular septic arthritis. Medicine (Baltimore) 1993;72(5):293–310.

Chlamydial arthritis

When Chlamydia is the suspected causative agent, patients may be given doxycycline or an analogue for up to 3 months, but optimal duration of therapy is unknown.[15]

OLIGOARTICULAR AND POLYARTICULAR NONINFECTIOUS ARTHRITIS

The term oligoarthritis refers to an inflammatory arthritis affecting 2 to 4 joints. It is the most common pattern seen among the seronegative arthropathies.[9] ReA

Table 3
Classification of polyarticular inflammatory joint disease

Symmetric Polyarticular	Asymmetric Oligoarticular
Infectious arthritis	Infectious arthritis
Viral	Gonococcal or meningococcal
Parvovirus	Lyme disease (late phase)
Hepatitis B and C	Fungal and mycobacterium
Others: HIV, EBV, rubella	Bacterial endocarditis
	Whipple disease
Postinfectious or reactive arthritic	Postinfectious or reactive arthritic
Rheumatic fever	Rheumatic fever
Poststreptococcal arthritis	Poststreptococcal arthritis
	ReA
	(Enteric, urogenital)
Palindromic rheumatism	Enteropathic arthritis of IBD
Juvenile idiopathic arthritis (polyarticular)	Juvenile idiopathic arthritis (polyarticular)
RA	Undifferentiated spondyloarthritis
PsA	PsA
Systemic rheumatic disease	Systemic rheumatic disease
Systemic lupus erythromatosus	Relapsing polychondritis
Sjögren sclerosis	Behçet disease
Systemic sclerosis	Crystal induced
Polymyositis or dermatomyositis	Gout
Mixed connective tissue disease	Pseudogout (calcium pyrophosphate
	deposition disease)
Still disease (juvenile, adult)	Basic calcium phosphate
Relapsing seronegative symmetrical	Other systemic illnesses
synovitis with pitting edema	
Polymyalgia rheumatica	Familial Mediterranean fever
Systemic vasculitis	Carcinomatous
Relapsing polychondritis	Pancreatic disease–associated arthritis
	Hyperlipoproteinemia
	Sarcoidosis (chronic)
	Multicentric reticulohistiocytosis
Other systemic illnesses	
Celiac disease	
Sarcoidosis (acute type)	
Acute leukemia (children)	
Peripheral arthritis with axial involvement	
Ankylosing spondylitis	
Enteropathic arthritis associated with IBD	
PsA	
ReA (enteric, urogenital)	
SAPHO (synovitis, acne, pustulosis,	
hyperostosis, osteitis)	
Whipple disease	

Abbreviations: EBV, Epstein-Barr virus; HIV, human immunodeficiency virus.

From West S. Musculoskeletal signs and symptoms. B. Polyarticular joint disease. In: Stone JH, Crofford LJ, editors. Primer on the rheumatic diseases. 13th edition. New York: Springer; 2008. p. 47–57; with permission.

(occasionally referred to as postinfectious arthritis), PsA, the arthritis associated with IBD, and SA are examples. Compared with polyarthritis, oligoarthritis typically affects younger people and generally has a better prognosis. A classification of the polyarticular inflammatory joint diseases is shown in **Table 4**.

DIAGNOSTIC APPROACH
History and Physical Examination

Acute polyarthritis, especially when accompanied by fever, is always caused by an inflammatory disease and requires immediate evaluation because infection or

Table 4
Suggestions for laboratory and imaging interventions that may support the diagnosis for selected diseases characterized primarily by polyarthritis

Possible Diagnosis	Clinical Constellation	Diagnostic Strategy
RA	Symmetric joint involvement, morning stiffness, anemia, serositis	RF, anti-CCP antibodies, ESR, CRP, CBC, radiograph of affected joints
SLE	Facial malar rash, photosensitivity, painless oral ulcers, serositis, seizure or psychosis in the absence of other causes	ANA, anti-ds DNA, anti-Sm, complement (C3,C4,CH50)
Ankylosing Spondylitis	Progressive stiffness of the spine in a young adult	Spinal radiograph, HLA-B27
Sjögren Syndrome	Parotid gland enlargement, lymphadenopathy, dryness of eyes, mouth mucosal ulceration	ANA, anti-Ro (anti-SSA), anti-La (anti-SSB)
ReA	Keratoderma blennorrhagicum, circinate balanitis, conjunctivitis	Screening for gonococcus or *Chlamydia trachomatis*, HLA-B27
PsA	Silvery skin plaques on extensor surfaces, involvement of DIP joints	Skin biopsy
Lyme Disease	Erythema migrans, bilateral Bell palsy, heart block	IgM and IgG antibodies to *Borrelia burgdoferi*, ECG
Sarcoidosis	Erythema nodosum, bilateral ankle arthritis, lymphadenopathy, scleritis	Chest radiograph, CBC, serum ACE level, lymph node biopsy
IBD	Abdominal pain with loose stools, perianal disease, weight loss, erythema nodosum, anemia	Colonoscopy
Drug-induced lupus	Discoid rash after recent medications like minocycline, hydralazine	ANA, antihistone antibodies

Abbreviations: ACE, angiotensin converting enzyme; ANA, antinuclear antibodies; Anti-CCP, antibodies to citrullinated proteins; Anti-dsDNA, antibodies to double-stranded DNA; CBC, complete blood cont; CRP, C-reactive protein; ECG, electrocardiogram; ESR, erythrocyte sedimentation rate; RF, rheumatoid factor.
Data from Fagan HB. Approach to the patient with acute swollen/painful joint. Clin Fam Pract 2005;7(2):305–19; Mathews CJ, Coakley G. Septic arthritis: current diagnosis and therapeutic algorithm. Curr Opin Rheumatol 2008;20:457–62; and Salzman BE, Nevin JE, Newman JH, et al. A primary care approach to the use and interpretation of common rheumatologic tests. Clin Fam Pract 2005;7(2):335–58.

crystalline arthritis can cause significant morbidity if left untreated. After taking a history, all joints should be carefully examined and the involved joints documented.

Pattern of joint involvement
Recruitment of newly affected joints while previously involved joints remain involved in the disease process is commonly seen in RA and other systemic rheumatic diseases. A migratory pattern, which refers to signs and symptoms being present in certain joints for a few days and then remitting, only to reappear in other joints, is most characteristic of rheumatic fever and occasionally gonorrhea.

Distribution of joint involvement
The most common cause of a chronic inflammatory polyarthritis that involves small and large joints bilaterally and symmetrically in the upper and lower extremities is RA. Inflammatory arthritis in an RA pattern also involving the distal interphalangeal joints of the fingers suggests PsA.

Associated extra-articular signs and symptoms and medical conditions
The presence of past or current extra-articular manifestations may provide important clues to the cause. For example, the presence of skin manifestations may suggest PsA. The presence of a pathognomonic rash might suggest Lyme disease, SLE, or rheumatic fever. The presence of oral ulcers might suggest Behçet disease. A history of injection drug use might suggest an infection with one of the causative agents of viral hepatitis. The use of medications such as hydralazine might suggest an iatrogenic cause. Additional clues might include pitting nails (PsA), keratoderma blennorrhagicum and circinate balanitis (ReA), lymphadenopathy, parotid enlargement, and dry eyes (Sjögren syndrome).

Patient demographics
Age is a helpful clue. Pseudogout is most common in older patients, and PsA, ReA, and ankylosing spondylitis are common in young people. Premenopausal women are 9 times more likely to develop SLE and 3 to 4 times more likely to develop RA. Polymyalgia rheumatica and Wegener granulomatosis are more likely to affect Caucasians, whereas sarcoidosis and SLE are more common in African Americans.

Laboratory Tests

Synovial fluid analysis
As mentioned previously, synovial fluid analysis should be performed in the febrile patient with an acute flare of established arthritis to rule out superimposed infectious arthritis.

Additional diagnostic testing (blood chemistry analysis, urinalysis, hematologic studies) should be ordered based on clinical suspicion. Serologic testing for markers of inflammation (erythrocyte sedimentation rate, C-reactive protein level) is a good starting point if an inflammatory process is suspected, although the positive predictive value of such tests is poor. More specific diagnostic tests (antinuclear antibody, rheumatoid factor, serologic titers) should be ordered based on clinical suspicion and the results of the screening evaluation. **Table 4** identifies a strategy based on the clinical suspicion and the results of screening studies.

MANAGEMENT OF NONINFECTIOUS INFLAMMATORY ARTHRITIS

Nonpharmacologic management is an important adjunct to drug therapy. Interventions include patient education, outpatient physical therapy, a home exercise program (including spinal extension exercises), and proper posturing. Inpatient rehabilitation may be necessary in selected patients.[15]

Treatment: First-Line Therapy (Mild to Moderate Severity)

NSAIDs

NSAIDs are effective in many inflammatory arthropathies and form the mainstay of drug treatment. These drugs must be used regularly to achieve the maximum analgesic and antiinflammatory effect. No definitive drug of choice has been identified, and the response to the drugs and degree of response vary among individuals.

NSAIDs have significant gastrointestinal, renal, and cardiovascular side effects. All individuals should be assessed, and a cyclooxygenase (COX) 2 selective drug should be used for those at high risk of upper gastrointestinal complications, such as gastrointestinal bleeding. Adding gastroprotective agents, such as misoprostol, H_2 receptor antagonists, or a proton pump inhibitor, to nonselective NSAIDs can reduce the risk of gastrointestinal complications. COX-2 selective drugs produce fewer gastrointestinal complications than COX-1 nonselective NSAIDs; however, the long-term use of COX-2 agents has been linked with a greater cardiovascular risk than that of COX-1 agents. Therefore, treatment should be given for the shortest period possible or avoided in at-risk patients.

Intra-articular corticosteroids

Intra-articular administration of corticosteroids has the advantage of delivering a high concentration of the agent to the involved joints and minimizing systemic adverse events caused by the drug. As an inflammatory oligoarthritis has the potential to evolve into a persistent polyarticular disease such as RA, which in turn can lead to irreversible joint damage, prompt and aggressive intervention can be disease modifying.[10]

Treatment: Second-Line Therapy (Moderate to Severe Severity Arthritis or Failure of First-Line Therapy)

Systemically administered corticosteroids

Corticosteroids, either as a short course of oral prednisone or as a single intramuscular dose of depot methylprednisolone, are valuable when severe symptoms arise from several joints, often in the presence of a constitutional illness. Patients who are required to use steroids on a long-term (more than 3 months) should be screened for osteoporosis and placed on an osteoporosis prevention program of exercise and calcium and vitamin D supplementation.

Biologic response modifiers

The NSAIDS and corticosteroids effectively relieve the inflammation and pain of arthritis, but do not alter the progression or the course of noninfectious inflammatory arthritis. The immunosuppressive agents, on the other hand, have anti-inflammatory activity and alter progression of these diseases. These medications (disease-modifying antirheumatic drugs [DMARDS] and immunosuppressive monoclonal antibodies) are used in consultation with the rheumatologist.

- The DMARDs comprise a series of antimetabolite and/or cytotoxic agents that include drugs such as azathioprine, gold compounds, hydroxyurea, methotrexate, penicillamine, and sulfasalazine.
- The immunosuppressive monoclonal antibodies represent a class of biologic response modifiers (BRMs) that include agents that bind and/or render tumor necrosis factor (TNF) ineffective (eg, etanercept, inflixamab, and the newer agent adalimumab or an agent that binds to CD80 and CD86 receptors on

antigen-presenting cells, which prevents the activation of selected T cells that promote or enhance inflammation [eg, abatacept, a more recently Food and Drug Administration–approved intravenously administered entity for RA]).

DMARDs (BRMs) are indicated when disabling symptoms persist for 3 or more months or evidence of erosive joint damage is present. Each of these drugs or biologic agents has its own toxicity that must be carefully monitored. For example, oral folic acid must be administered to patients who are on the folate reductase inhibitor, methotrexate. Patients who are given TNF inhibitors must be monitored for infusion reactions, an increased risk of infection including tuberculosis, development of autoantibodies, SLE, vasculitis, demyelinating disease, and worsening congestive heart failure.

Additional Comments on Specific Arthritides

ReA
Symptomatic treatment is accomplished with high doses of selected NSAIDs, such as indomethacin (25–50 mg 3 times a day). Oral corticosteroids are not as effective, but intra-articular steroid injections in patients with large knee effusions can be helpful.[10,15] In another study of patients with ReA following a recurrent episode of urethritis, erythromycin or tetracycline therapy (500 mg 4 times a day) limited recurrences to 10%. Patients with persistent signs and symptoms can be treated with sulfasalazine, 1 to 3 g, given orally once daily. In patients who develop deformities or who show radiographic evidence of erosions or sacroiliitis, methotrexate and azathioprine have been shown to be helpful. These 2 medications should not be used in patients suspected to be infected with HIV.[15]

Ankylosing spondylitis
Treatment of ankylosing spondylitis begins with an NSAID. A positive response to NSAID therapy is actually helpful in diagnosing ankylosing spondylitis. Oral corticosteroids in conventional dosages are of little value in the treatment of ankylosing spondylitis, but intra-articular corticosteroid injections can provide rapid and sustained relief in isolated inflamed joints.[10] Second-line agents, such as sulfasalazine, are used when patients do not respond to or are unable to tolerate NSAIDs.

PsA
Treatment of PsA is directed at both the skin and joint manifestations. A variety of topical therapies, including corticosteroids, retinoids, and ultraviolet light therapy, can be used for the skin disease. NSAID therapy, the initial treatment for joint manifestations, improves swelling and tenderness. Intra-articular corticosteroid injections usually control localized joint disease, but oral corticosteroid therapy may occasionally be needed in the treatment of more generalized disease. Second-line agents include methotrexate, sulfasalazine, cyclosporine, and TNF-α inhibitors and are used in consultation with the rheumatologist.

IBD arthropathy
NSAIDs should be used cautiously, because they can exacerbate the bowel disease. Sulfasalazine has been effective in the treatment of IBD and arthritis.

Indications for referral Appropriate and timely referral to the appropriate specialist, when indicated, is also part of the prudent management of the patient with joint pain with the following conditions[3]:

- Suspected infectious arthritis with sepsis
- Undiagnosed multisystem or systemic rheumatic disease

- Undiagnosed synovitis, in which arthrocentesis or synovial biopsy may be needed
- Musculoskeletal pain undiagnosed after 6 weeks
- Unexplained immunochemical test result abnormalities suggestive of an underlying rheumatic disease
- Musculoskeletal pain not adequately controlled with therapy
- Musculoskeletal pain associated with severe or progressive loss of function or work productivity
- Conditions for which treatment with steroids or immunosuppressive drugs is considered
- Systemic rheumatic disease in a pregnant or postpartum patient.

A timely referral for consultation with a rheumatologist is likely to be far more productive than exhaustive serologic testing, with its high risk of false-positive results and attendant adverse consequences, and excessive use of imaging techniques, especially CT and MRI.

SUMMARY

Joint pain is a common complaint that patients present with in a busy primary care office. A thorough history, with special attention to risk factors, physical examination, and synovial fluid analysis, is the most important aspect in the care of these patients. A well-trained and experienced primary care physician can arrive at the right diagnosis by paying attention to the patient's diagnostic clues (eg, young patients who present with fever, joint pain, and genital discharge; middle-aged patients who present with acute joint pain following a bout of alcohol use; women with skin rash and photosensitivity; and young men with bloody diarrhea, abdominal pain, and painful, swollen joints).

REFERENCES

1. Centers for Disease Control and Prevention. Prevalance of disabilities and associated health conditions among adults: United States 1999. Morb Mortal Wkly Rep 2001;50:120–5.
2. Stange KC, Zyzananski SJ, Jaen CR, et al. Illuminating the "black box". A description of 4454 patient visits to 138 to family physicians. J Fam Pract 1998;46(5):377–89.
3. Ho G Jr. Infectious disorders. In: Klippel JH, Stone JH, Crofford LJ, et al, editors. Primer on the rheumatic diseases. 13th edition. New York: Springer Science; 2008. p. 271–6.
4. Fagan HB. Approach to the patient with acute swollen/painful joint. Clin Fam Pract 2005;7(2):305–19.
5. Mathews CJ, Coakley G. Septic arthritis: current diagnosis and therapeutic algorithm. Curr Opin Rheumatol 2008;20:457–62.
6. Garcia-De LaTorre I. Gonococcal and nongonococcal arthritis. Rheum Dis Clin North Am 2009;35:63–73.
7. Schmerling RH, Fuchs HA, Lorish CD, et al. American College of Rheumatology Adhoc Committee on Clinical Guidelines. Guidelines for the initial evaluation of the adult patient with acute musculoskeletal symptoms. Arthritis Rheum 1996; 39(1):1–8.
8. Marzo-Ortega H. Early oligoarthritis. Rheum Dis Clin North Am 2005;31:627–39.

9. Coakley G, Mathews CJ, Field M, et al. BSR& BHPR, BOA, RCGP and BSAC guidelines for the management of the hot swollen joint in adults. Rheumatology (Oxford) 2006;45:1039–41.
10. Kaandorp CJE, Kriknen P, Moens HJB, et al. The outcome of bacterial arthritis. A prospective community-based study. Arthritis Rheum 1997;40(5):884–92.
11. Dubost JJ, Fis I, Denis P, et al. Polyarticular septic arthritis. Medicine (Baltimore) 1993;72(5):293–310.
12. Barth WF, Segal K. Reactive arthritis (Reiter's syndrome). Am Fam Physician 1999;60(2):499–510.
13. Barth WF. Office evaluation of the patient with musculoskeletal complaints. Am J Med 1997;102:3–10.
14. Salzman BE, Nevin JE, Newman JH, et al. A primary care approach to the use and interpretation of common rheumatologic tests. Clin Fam Pract 2005;7(2): 335–58.
15. Bardin T, Enel C, Cornelis F, et al. Antibiotic treatment of venereal disease and Reiter's syndrome in a Greenland population. Arthritis Rheum 1992;35(2):190–4.

.

Low Back Pain: An Approach to Diagnosis and Management

R. Lamar Duffy, MD

KEYWORDS

• Lumbar • Back • Pain • Sciatica • Lumbago

Low back pain is one of the top 10 problems prompting a visit to a family physician.[1] Low back pain afflicts both sexes equally, with a peak onset at age 30 to 40 years and a lifetime incidence as high as 85%.[2,3] Although two-thirds of cases of back pain resolve within 6 weeks, it is the most common and most expensive cause of work-related disability in the population younger than 45 years.[4] Direct medical costs due to low back pain in the United States have been estimated at $12.2 to $90.6 billion per year; this may represent only about 15% of the total cost to society, with lost productivity and disability compensation drastically increasing the final sum.[3,5] Thus there is clear need for evidence-based guidance regarding low back pain management, the bulk of which is provided by primary care physicians.[6]

DIAGNOSIS
Definitions and Differential Diagnosis

Low back pain is pain localized to the lumbar area between the inferior ribcage and the waistline, though it may include sciatica, with pain radiating down the posterior-lateral thigh distal to the knee. It has commonly been divided by duration into acute (<6 weeks), subacute (6 to 12 weeks), and chronic (longer than 12 weeks). The majority of patients with acute low back pain experience spontaneous resolution within a month[1] and will not seek medical care.[2]

When patients do present with low back pain, the practitioner must be aware of the most common causes, while being attentive to "red flags" that indicate more serious conditions. To that end, while the etiology of low back pain may be categorized in several ways, it is helpful for the clinician to think in terms of 4 general causes: nonspecific, mechanical, nonmechanical, and referred visceral. **Table 1** lists examples and

Financial support: None.

Department of Family Medicine, University of South Alabama, 1504 Springhill Avenue, Suite 3414, Mobile, AL 36604, USA

E-mail address: rlduffy@usouthal.edu

doi:10.1016/j.pop.2010.07.003
primarycare.theclinics.com

Key Points	
Recommendation	Level of Evidence
Evaluation	
In the absence of red flags, diagnostic imaging should be deferred in favor of 4–6 weeks of conservative care	C
Patients with persistent low back pain and signs of radiculopathy or spinal stenosis unresponsive to conservative therapy should be evaluated with MRI (preferred) or CT only if they are candidates for surgery or epidural steroid injection	B
Recognition of psychosocial yellow flags is useful in identification of patients with a poor prognosis	B
Treatment	
Bed rest is not effective, and bed rest exceeding 2–3 days may be harmful; patients should be advised to remain active	A
Acetaminophen and NSAIDs are effective first-line medications for acute or chronic low back pain	A
Skeletal muscle relaxants are effective for short-term pain relief in patients who tolerate them	A
Tricyclic antidepressants are effective for chronic low back pain in patients who tolerate them	B
For patients not responding to initial therapy, heat, spinal manipulation, acupuncture, massage, education, exercise, and multidisciplinary/behavioral measures offer therapeutic value	B

relative distributions of these categories. Although many patients with nonspecific "low back sprains" self-manage the problem, nonspecific back pain still represents 70% of the cases that present to a physician, regardless of the acute-to-chronic timing.[2,4,6]

Red and Yellow Flags

Red flags are findings suggesting the need for immediate surgical attention, or indicative of important underlying conditions such as infection or malignancy. The use of flags to direct imaging strategy is an approach that has been standard since 1994.[7,8] A commonly used red flag list is given in **Table 2**. Knowledge of these indicators allows the physician to reduce the usage of unnecessary and expensive diagnostic testing in the majority of patients for which they will be noncontributory, while highlighting those patients most likely to have a complicated course.

Psychosocial barriers to recovery, which indicate a protracted course and poorer prognosis, are important to recognize as well. These "yellow flags" are a combination of behaviors, beliefs, work history, social factors, and affective symptoms that do not lend themselves to as neat a "check list" as the red flags, yet are intuitive to most physicians who care for patients with back pain. One collection of yellow flags is given in **Table 3**. While not particularly altering the initial evaluation, yellow flags have

Table 1	
Differential diagnosis of low back pain [percentage of adult low back pain patients in primary care]	
Nonspecific (70%)	Lumbar sprain/strain [70%]
Mechanical (27%)	Degenerative disc/facet disease [10%]
	Herniated disc [4%]
	Osteoporotic fracture, usually compression[a] [4%]
	Spinal stenosis [3%]
	Spondylolisthesis [2%]
	Traumatic fracture[a]
	Congenital disease (severe kyphosis, scoliosis, transitional vertebrae)
	Other[b] (spondylosis, internal disc disruption, presumed instability)
Visceral/referred, nonmalignant (2%)	Aortic aneurysm
	Pelvic organ diseases (prostatitis, endometriosis, pelvic inflammatory disease)
	Gastrointestinal disease (pancreatitis, cholecystitis, penetrating peptic ulcer)
	Renal disease (nephrolithiasis, pyelonephritis)[a]
Nonmechanical (1%)	Neoplasia (multiple myeloma, metastatic carcinoma, lymphoma, leukemia, spinal cord tumors, retroperitoneal tumors, primary vertebral tumors)
	Inflammatory arthritis, often HLA-B27-positive (ankylosing spondylitis, psoriatic spondylitis, Reiter syndrome, inflammatory bowel disease)
	Infection (osteomyelitis, septic discitis, paraspinous abscess, epidural abscess, perinephric abscess, shingles)[a]
	Scheuermann disease (osteochondrosis)
	Paget disease of bone

Conditions without percentages listed account for <1% of low back pain.
[a] More likely to present as acute pain.
[b] Conditions often seen in normal patients, or controversial/inconsistently-defined conditions.
Data from Refs.[2,4,6]

implications with regard to therapeutic choices and realistic expectations, and thus are useful at early encounters with low back pain patients.[6,9–11]

History

An experienced clinician will be able to rapidly obtain a targeted history, identify red or yellow flags, and determine the likelihood of serious illness. Basic demographic information and a description of the present illness is important, with attention to review of medications and systemic gynecologic, urinary, gastrointestinal, rheumatologic, and neoplastic diseases. A history of prior back pain, osteoporosis, injury, or temporal relationship with activity is informative, as is a review of systems including unexplained fever, weight loss, nighttime pain, and substance abuse. A survey of the psychosocial yellow flags should be undertaken in a diplomatic fashion that avoids putting the patient in the position of immediately having to defend the legitimacy of his or her pain.[4,6]

Physical Examination

Physical examination begins with the collection of vital signs and a systemic survey aimed at identifying evidence of nonmechanical and visceral causes of low back pain. Focus is then shifted to localization of the pain, with examination by inspection,

Table 2
Red flags for low back pain, and associated diagnoses of concern

	Cauda Equina Syndrome	Fracture	Malignancy	Infection
Age >70		X	X	
Minor trauma with age >50		X	X	
Significant trauma		X		
Unexplained fever				X
Recent urinary infection; skin infection or penetrating wound near spine				X
Unrelenting night or rest pain			X	X
Progressive or disabling neurologic deficit (saddle anesthesia, bilateral sciatica, bilateral leg weakness, difficulty voiding, fecal incontinence)	X		X	
Unexplained weight loss			X	
History or strong suspicion of cancer			X	
Osteoporosis		X		
Chronic steroid use		X		X
Immunosuppression				X
Intravenous drug abuse				X
Lack of improvement after 6 weeks of conservative therapy			X	X

Data from Kinkade S. Evaluation and treatment of acute low back pain. Am Fam Physician 2007;75:1181–8, 1190–2; and Bradley WG, Seidenwurm DJ, Brunberg JA, et al, for the American College of Radiology. ACR appropriateness criteria: low back pain. Available at: http://www.acr.org/SecondaryMainMenuCategories/quality_safety/app_criteria/pdf/ExpertPanelonNeurologicImaging/LowBackPainDoc7.aspx. Accessed September 4, 2009.

palpation, and percussion. Radiation of pain should be noted, along with deformity suggestive of degenerative disease or osteoporotic fractures.

As several of the red flags and more common mechanical causes of low back pain are indicated by motor or sensory deficits, the neurologic examination often becomes the primary focus. Neurologic findings consistent with cauda equina syndrome, including saddle anesthesia, bilateral radiculopathy, bilateral leg weakness, urinary retention and overflow incontinence, and fecal incontinence require immediate referral. Without neurologic deficit, pain localized to the lumbar spine and buttocks is more commonly seen in lumbar strains and degenerative disease. Limitation of spinal range of motion is a nonspecific finding that is not strongly associated with any particular diagnosis.[2,4]

Significant disc herniation may lead to nerve root impingement, resulting in sciatica. Such pain radiates below the level of the knee, and is often aggravated by Valsalva maneuvers.[2,4] While only about 4% of low back pain patients have a herniated disc, 95% of those with a herniation experience sciatica, so its absence rules out a herniated disc to a high degree of certainty.[2] Approximately 95% of lumbar disc herniations involve the L5 and S1 nerve roots. A rapid assessment of the L4, L5, and S1 nerve roots can be accomplished by testing sensation of the medial, dorsal, and lateral foot, respectively; a motor assessment of the same respective roots is done by having the patient stand from squatting, heel-walk, and toe-walk. Diminished deep tendon reflexes may also be demonstrated.[2,4]

Table 3 Yellow flags for low back pain prognosis	
Affective	Depression and symptoms of depression
	Anxiety and symptoms of anxiety
	Irritability
Behavioral	Poor coping skills
	Impaired or excessive sleep
	Passive attitude about and poor compliance with rehabilitation
	Dramatically reduced activities of daily living
	Social withdrawal
	Increased use of alcohol or other substances of abuse
Belief	Catastrophic thinking
	Belief that pain is uncontrollable
	Belief that pain is physically harmful
	Belief that pain must be completely eliminated before returning to work
	Misinterpretation/exaggeration of other somatic symptoms
	Expectation of a technological solution for back pain
Social	Lack of support system
	Overprotective family/friends
	Socially punitive family/friends
	Low educational background
	History of physical, sexual, or substance abuse
Occupational	Expectation of worsening pain or setbacks with activity
	Poor work history, frequent lost time
	Poor job satisfaction
	Unsupportive work environment
	Problems with claims and compensation
	Pending litigation

Data from Refs.[6,9–11]

The most commonly used test of lumbar disc herniation is straight leg raising, whereby the patient is placed supine, with the examiner passively flexing the thigh while maintaining knee extension. A positive test is pain radiating below the knee on thigh flexion between 30° and 60° to 75°,[6,12] though some maintain that pain at any degree of flexion is notable, with pain brought on by lesser degrees of flexion indicating more severe disease.[13] Both legs should be tested, as there are different implications when pain appears in the same or opposite leg. Studies have revealed 91% sensitivity and 26% specificity for lumbar disc herniation when pain is elicited on the side of the flexed thigh, with sensitivity and specificity of 29% and 88%, respectively, if pain appears in the opposite leg (the cross straight leg raising test).[12] In other words, if pain occurs on the same side as the flexed thigh, lumbar disc herniation is possible, but if pain is on the opposite side, herniation is more likely.

Diagnostic Testing

The prevalence of low back pain and the frequency of abnormal findings in asymptomatic patients present a significant opportunity to do more harm than good with diagnostic testing. Indiscriminate testing leads to unnecessary medical expense, which grows exponentially when incidentally discovered abnormalities generate further testing. Suspicious results cause anxiety for both patient and provider, and can inadvertently reinforce any yellow flags that may be present. Combined with the self-limited nature of most back pain, the clinician is obliged to be judicious with regard to diagnostic testing.

Laboratory evaluation for low back pain is of limited utility, and is focused on identification of visceral and nonmechanical diseases suggested by red flags. A complete blood count, erythrocyte sedimentation rate, and C-reactive protein, while nonspecific, would all be reasonable initial studies in the face of most any red flag other than trauma or osteoporosis, whereas a urinalysis would be indicated only if urologic disease were suspected. A prostate-specific antigen would be of value as a secondary test when evaluation suggests prostate cancer,[2,14] while alkaline phosphatase and calcium would be in order if there were clinical clues for metabolic bone disease.[6]

Radiographic imaging is the most commonly ordered study for low back pain. Patients with back pain often expect radiographs, and many clinicians take the path of least resistance by performing them. Yet there is uniform agreement that in the absence of red flags, diagnostic imaging is not warranted unless 4 to 6 weeks of conservative management have failed to achieve improvement.[2,4,6–8,15–17] It is the responsibility of the physician to explain that in uncomplicated cases of low back pain radiography is not helpful, and may, in fact, be counterproductive. Imaging also serves little purpose if no therapeutic decision will be affected by the result.

Plain radiography, computed tomography (CT), and magnetic resonance imaging (MRI) are the studies most likely to be ordered by primary care physicians. Although plain radiography has the advantage of low cost and ready availability, it is compromised by being minimally useful in evaluating soft tissue. Traumatic fracture can be identified, but will often require more extensive evaluation for definitive diagnosis; proceeding directly to more advanced imaging, if rapidly available, may be logical when suspicion of fracture is high. Compression fracture may be detected, but it is difficult to distinguish acute from chronic compression with plain films. Degenerative changes such as spurring may be detected, but these findings are common with aging, and often asymptomatic. Plain radiography usually only displays evidence of other systemic red flags at later stages of the clinical course.[18]

CT is now almost universally available, and can often be performed on an urgent basis. CT scans excel at detecting traumatic and degenerative changes in cortical bone, and have been shown to have similar sensitivity and specificity as MRI in detecting herniated discs.[19] CT can demonstrate foraminal and extraforaminal nerve root impingement, and is superior to plain films in detecting infection and neoplasm.[4,18]

Compared with CT, MRI provides superior soft tissue detail. While overall sensitivity and specificity for disc disease is similar to CT, the added detail may help in separating symptomatic disc extrusion from incidentally detected bulging. MRI is the method of choice for detecting malignancy and infection in the spine, provides better visualization of intrathecal nerve roots and bone marrow, and requires no radiation. Disadvantages include higher cost, lower availability, longer testing time,[18] and the risk of nephrogenic systemic fibrosis associated with gadolinium contrast in patients with compromised renal function.[20] MRI is inferior to CT in visualization of cortical bone, and thus has less utility in the setting of acute fracture.[18]

A major pitfall of all methods of imaging is the high rate of abnormal findings in asymptomatic people. In a review of MRI of asymptomatic adults, herniated discs were discovered in 9% to 76% of patients, with bulging discs (20%–81%), degenerative discs (46%–93%), annular disc tears (14%–56%), and spinal stenosis (1%–21%) also appearing as frequent findings. Against this backdrop, it is imperative for the clinician to be selective in the performance of radiographic studies, as guided by the clinical setting and red flags.[2,18]

MANAGEMENT

Treatment of low back pain is often tinted with unrealistic expectations on the part of the patient, family, employer, and even medical providers. Guided by red flags, the physician should rapidly identify problems that require urgent intervention. Beyond that, a respectful adherence to the "first, do no harm" axiom is in order. Initial treatment is aimed at providing comfort, while the focus soon turns to the resumption of normal activities.

Surgery

Red flags may reveal the presence of cauda equina syndrome, which demands rapid surgical decompression, or nonspinal/systemic processes such as aortic aneurysm, infection, or neoplasm, that have either definitive or palliative treatment. However, there is virtually no role for surgery in patients with nonspecific low back pain, and most patients displaying radiculopathy will also improve without surgery. In the presence of fracture, infection, progressive deformity, or spondylolisthesis leading to instability, there is supportive evidence for spinal fusion.[21] Decompression is sometimes performed for degenerative disc disease and spondylosis; while innovative procedures are being developed for such indications the results are conflicting, and improvement is often short-lived.[4,6,22] Nonetheless, in patients who have significant disability and pain despite a year of conservative therapy, and who have anatomic pathology consistent with their symptoms, decompressive surgery is a reasonable option.[6]

Pharmacologic Treatment

Most studies of medications have been in the setting of nonspecific low back pain, or in mixed populations of patients with acute or chronic pain, with or without radicular components. The most definitive evidence supports short-term improvement in pain, whereas long-term benefit for chronic pain is more nebulous and is coupled with increased risk of side effects. It is thus prudent to use analgesics for the shortest duration necessary, stopping when continued benefit is no longer clearly appreciated.[16]

There is strong evidence that nonsteroidal anti-inflammatory drugs (NSAIDs) are superior to placebo for acute low back pain, with more modest data for chronic pain.[2,6,16,23] Cyclooxygenase-2 inhibitors are no more effective than conventional NSAIDs.[23,24] Use of NSAIDs must be weighed against their known risks of gastrointestinal and renal toxicity, along with recently raised questions about increased risk of myocardial infarction. There are insufficient data for or against the use of aspirin for back pain.[16]

There are conflicting data as to whether acetaminophen is equivalent, or slightly inferior, to NSAIDs for the treatment of low back pain.[6,16,25] Acetaminophen avoids the renal and gastrointestinal risks of NSAIDs, though there is the specter of hepatotoxicity, given the ease with which inadvertent overdose may occur. Still, its overall favorable safety profile makes it a reasonable first-line treatment.

Although there is a question about the role of muscle spasm in low back pain, muscle relaxants are superior to placebo for short-term pain relief. Drawbacks to muscle relaxants include their common side effects of sedation and dizziness, and for this reason they are not generally used for longer than 1 to 2 weeks. It should also be noted that benzodiazepines and carisoprodol (through its metabolism to meprobamate) carry significant risk of habituation and abuse.[2,16,26]

Tramadol, a weak opioid and serotonin-norepinephrine reuptake inhibitor, is effective for short-term relief of low back pain. While unscheduled in most states, it may cause sedation, constipation, and nausea, and should be avoided in recovering narcotic addicts. Still, it is a relatively safe alternative, capable of improving pain and activities of daily living.[6,25,27]

Opiates have a controversial role in the treatment of low back pain. While capable of providing potent, short-term pain relief, their side effects of sedation, constipation, and habituation make them less than ideal choices for long-term use, and there are few high-quality studies addressing their use in that setting. Some reviews have found no difference in short-term pain relief between narcotics and NSAIDs,[27] whereas others have demonstrated greater efficacy with long-term opioids for pain and mood than with NSAIDs.[28] Opiates have not been shown to improve activity levels[27,28] or facilitate return to work.[29] Narcotic analgesics are a reasonable second- or third-line choice for severe, acute back pain,[2] and may have a place in the setting of chronic pain management for patients with severely impaired quality of life and no surgically correctable pathology, but generally they are not appropriate for long-term management of low back pain.[4,16]

Tricyclic antidepressants are beneficial for chronic pain, and thus have value in the treatment of back pain for patients who are able to tolerate their sedating and anticholinergic effects.[4,6,16] Selective serotonin reuptake inhibitors (SSRIs), on the other hand, do not seem to be effective.[6,16] Some serotonin-norepinephrine reuptake inhibitors are approved for diabetic neuropathy and fibromyalgia, raising the question of utility in back pain,[30] though this potential has not yet been demonstrated.[6,16] It should be noted, however, that depression is often concomitant with chronic back pain, and in such cases any antidepressant may be therapeutic.

Several other medications are used in the management of chronic pain, and thus have been considered for back pain. Various anticonvulsants are sometimes cast in this role, though only gabapentin has clearly demonstrated efficacy, for patients with radiculopathy.[6,16] Pregabalin has also been used in a similar setting, though without supportive data. Systemic corticosteroids have been employed for acute low back pain, but there are no studies demonstrating benefit over placebo. Epidural steroid injections, on the other hand, have been shown to provide relief for patients displaying radicular symptoms, though the response is modest, individually variable, and temporary, lasting weeks to months.[2,16]

Nonpharmacologic Treatment

Evaluation of nonpharmacologic measures for low back pain is challenging. Therapies are employed in various manners by a broad assortment of disciplines. Studies are often small, of marginal quality, and hampered by the inherent difficulty in blinding presented by the treatments themselves. Choice of controls can be problematic against the background of spontaneous resolution often seen with back pain. Despite these issues, several nonmedicinal treatments are commonly used by patients, and some conclusions can be drawn from the literature.

Available evidence firmly attests to the lack of benefit of bed rest for low back pain. Extended bed rest may actually delay resolution of pain and resumption of normal activities, whether pain is nonspecific or sciatic, while immediate return to normal activities as tolerated is associated with rapid recovery.[2,4,24,31] Such return-to-work recommendations obviously require the cooperation of employers, and must take into account the physical demands of the patient's normal activities. Exclusive bed rest should be avoided under most circumstances, and if recommended should last no longer than 2 to 3 days. Patients need to be reassured that ongoing pain does not imply harm, and in fact, muscles that remain inactive may become hypersensitive to pain, prolonging disability.[4,6]

Studies regarding therapeutic exercise are conflicting. Most studies reveal that formal back exercises are not useful for acute back pain.[2,4,32,33] In chronic low back pain, back exercises may lead to small improvements in pain, function, time lost from work, and recurrence, though few reviews find such improvements to be statistically or clinically significant.[4,6,23,32,34]

Spinal manipulation is commonly used by patients for low back pain; as many as 45% of patients with back pain consult a chiropractor.[6] Studies of spinal manipulation are heterogeneous and procedurally difficult to design. Many reviews have found manipulation superior to placebo, though improvements are generally modest in magnitude and duration and are similar in efficacy to other conservative measures.[2,4,16,35,36] Lumbar spine manipulation is safe in the hands of an experienced practitioner, and benefits appear to be independent of the specific discipline of the provider.[2,6]

Acupuncture is also challenging to formally evaluate. Whereas some studies have shown efficacy superior to conventional therapy,[37] most report benefits in pain and function of brief duration and on par with other commonly used treatments.[2,6,38] Sham acupuncture often appears to convey similar benefits, raising questions about its mechanism of action and the contribution of nonspecific effects.[37,39,40] Nonetheless, given its safety, acupuncture may have a role alongside other conservative measures, especially if it reduces the need for higher-risk medications or procedures.

Several other pain management modalities are often employed for low back pain. There is modest evidence that heat provides short-term relief in both acute and chronic low back pain; cold packs may also be beneficial, though data are less abundant.[2,41] Massage is safe and often embraced by patients, though evidence of efficacy is better for subacute and chronic pain.[2,42] Lumbar traction does not appear to be useful for back pain, regardless of the presence of sciatica.[43] Several technical modalities have been used for the treatment of low back pain, including transcutaneous electrical nerve stimulation (TENS), ultrasonography, interferential therapy, low-level laser therapy, and shortwave diathermy, though there is little evidence of their utility.[44]

It is difficult to argue against education, though quality research on its impact is limited. Individual instruction addressing the importance of continued activity and fear of pain issues is useful; in fact, the educational component of the initial visit with a physical therapist provides much of the value of such consultations.[2,45] Educational media,[46] guided self-management programs,[47] and multidisciplinary rehabilitation programs that incorporate a cognitive-behavioral component all appear to convey some benefit, especially in vocational settings.[16,23]

SUMMARY

Low back pain is a very common condition, responsible for significant morbidity and economic impact on society. Although most cases spontaneously resolve, the clinician must be alert to red flags, such as fever, weight loss, advanced age, progressive neurologic deficit, osteoporosis, chronic steroid therapy, or substance abuse, which suggest the presence of systemic illness or imminent neurologic compromise in need of immediate and definitive treatment. In the absence of such findings, diagnostic imaging generally does not contribute to management, and may be safely delayed for 6 to 12 weeks. Continued activity as tolerated is associated with favorable outcomes. Acetaminophen, NSAIDs, muscle relaxants, and tricyclic antidepressants provide meaningful relief, whereas use of opiates should be limited to brief periods

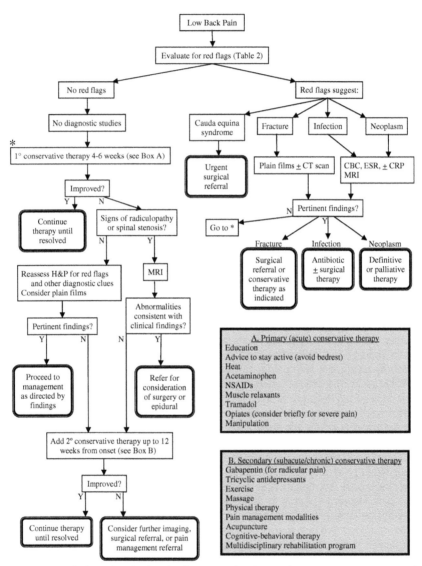

Fig. 1. Suggested algorithm for low back pain evaluation and management. CBC, complete blood count; CRP, C-reactive protein; ESR, erythrocyte sedimentation rate; H&P, history-taking and physical examination. (*Data from* Refs.[2,6,15,16])

for more severe pain. When pain becomes protracted, several nonpharmacologic measures may have utility in reducing pain and improving return to normal activities. **Fig. 1** presents an algorithm for the evaluation and management of low back pain.

REFERENCES

1. Bratton R. Assessment and management of acute low back pain. Am Fam Physician 1999;60:2299–308.

2. Kinkade S. Evaluation and treatment of acute low back pain. Am Fam Physician 2007;75:1181–8, 1190–2.
3. Haldeman S, Dagenais S. A supermarket approach to the evidence-informed management of chronic low back pain. Spine J 2008;8(1):1–7.
4. Deyo RA, Weinstein JN. Low back pain. N Engl J Med 2001;344(5):363–70.
5. Dagenais S, Caro J, Haldeman S. A systematic review of low back pain cost of illness studies in the United States and internationally. Spine J 2008;8(1):8–20.
6. Last A, Hulbert K. Chronic low back pain: evaluation and management. Am Fam Physician 2009;79(12):1067–74.
7. Bigos SJ, Bowyer OR, Braen GR, et al. Acute low back problems in adults. Clinical practice guideline no. 14 (AHCPR publication no. 95-0642). Rockville (MD): U.S. Department of Health and Human Services, Public Health Service, Agency for Health Care Policy and Research; 1994.
8. Bradley WG, Seidenwurm DJ, Brunberg JA, et al, for the American College of Radiology. ACR appropriateness criteria: low back pain. Available at: http://www.acr.org/SecondaryMainMenuCategories/quality_safety/app_criteria/pdf/ExpertPanelonNeurologicImaging/LowBackPainDoc7.aspx. Accessed September 4, 2009.
9. Mallen CD, Peat G, Thomas E, et al. Prognostic factors for musculoskeletal pain in primary care: a systematic review. Br J Gen Pract 2007;57(541):655–61.
10. New Zealand Guidelines Group. New Zealand acute low back pain guide. Wellington, New Zealand. 2004. Available at: http://www.nzgg.org.nz/guidelines/0072/acc1038_col.pdf. Accessed September 2, 2009.
11. Jensen S. Back pain—clinical assessment. Aust Fam Physician 2004;33(6):393–401.
12. Devillé WL, van der Windt DA, Dzaferagic A, et al. The test of Lasègue: systematic review of the accuracy in diagnosing herniated discs. Spine 2000;25(9):1140–7.
13. Jönsson B, Strömqvist B. The straight leg raising test and the severity of symptoms in lumbar disc herniation. A preoperative evaluation. Spine (Phila Pa 1976). 1995;20(1):27–30.
14. Malmivaara A. Low back pain. Article ID: ebm00435 (020.030), © 2007 Duodecim Medical Publications Ltd. Available at: http://www.essentialevidenceplus.com/content/index.cfm?request_path=/content/ebmg_ebm/435&. Accessed August 31, 2009.
15. Institute for Clinical Systems Improvement (ICSI). Adult low back pain. Bloomington (MN): Institute for Clinical Systems Improvement (ICSI); 2008. p. 66.
16. Chou R, Qaseem A, Snow V, et al, for the Clinical Efficacy Assessment Subcommittee of the American College of Physicians, American College of Physicians, American Pain Society Low Back Pain Guidelines Panel. Diagnosis and treatment of low back pain: a joint clinical practice guideline from the American College of Physicians and the American Pain Society. Ann Intern Med 2007;147(7):478–91.
17. Hegmann KT. Low back disorders. In: Glass LS, editor. Occupational medicine practice guidelines: evaluation and management of common health problems and functional recovery in workers. 2nd edition. Elk Grove Village (IL): American College of Occupational and Environmental Medicine (ACOEM); 2007. p. 366.
18. Jarvik JG, Deyo RA. Diagnostic evaluation of low back pain with emphasis on imaging. Ann Intern Med 2002;137:586–97.
19. Thornbury JR, Fryback DG, Turski PA, et al. Disk-caused nerve compression in patients with acute low-back pain: diagnosis with MR, CT myelography, and plain CT. Radiology 1993;186:731–8.

20. Wertman R, Altun E, Martin DR, et al. Risk of nephrogenic systemic fibrosis: evaluation of gadolinium chelate contrast agents at four American universities. Radiology 2008;248:799–806.
21. Don AS, Carragee E. A brief overview of evidence-informed management of chronic low back pain with surgery. Spine J 2008;8(1):258–65.
22. Gibson JN, Waddell G. Surgery for degenerative lumbar spondylosis. Cochrane Database Syst Rev 2005;4:CD001352.
23. van Tulder MW, Koes BW, Bouter LM. Conservative treatment of acute and chronic nonspecific low back pain: a systematic review of randomized controlled trials of the most common interventions. Spine 1997;22:2128–56.
24. Michigan Quality Improvement Consortium. Management of acute low back pain. Southfield (MI): Michigan Quality Improvement Consortium; 2008. p. 11.
25. Ruoff GE, Rosenthal N, Jordan D, et al. Tramadol/acetaminophen combination tablets for the treatment of chronic lower back pain: a multicenter, randomized, double-blind, placebo-controlled outpatient study. Clin Ther 2003;25(4): 1123–41.
26. van Tulder MW, Touray T, Furlan AD, et al. Muscle relaxants for non-specific low back pain. Cochrane Database Syst Rev 2003;2:CD004252.
27. Deshpande A, Furlan A, Mailis-Gagnon A, et al. Opioids for chronic low-back pain. Cochrane Database Syst Rev 2007;3:CD004959.
28. Jamison RN, Raymond SA, Slawsby EA, et al. Opioid therapy for chronic non-cancer back pain: a randomized prospective study. Spine 1998;23:2591–600.
29. van Tulder MW, Scholten RJ, Koes BW, et al. Nonsteroidal antiinflammatory drugs for low back pain. Cochrane Database Syst Rev 2006;2:CD000396.
30. Arehart-Treichel Joan. Antidepressants show promise in pain management. Psychiatr News 2006;41:30–1.
31. Hagen KB, Hilde G, Jamtvedt G, et al. Bed rest for acute low-back pain and sciatica. Cochrane Database Syst Rev 2004;4:CD001254.
32. Hayden JA, van Tulder MW, Malmivaara A, et al. Exercise therapy for treatment of non-specific low back pain. Cochrane Database Syst Rev 2005;3:CD000335.
33. Kukkonen-Harjula K, Vuori I, Finnish Medical Society Duodecim. Physical activity in the prevention, treatment and rehabilitation of diseases. In: Kukkonen-Harjula K, Vuori I, editors. EBM Guidelines. Evidence-based medicine [Internet]. Helsinki (Finland): Wiley Interscience. John Wiley & Sons; 2007 [Various].
34. Carter IR, Lord JL. Clinical inquiries. How effective are exercise and physical therapy for chronic low back pain? J Fam Pract 2002;51(3):209.
35. Assendelft WJJ, Morton SC, Yu EI, et al. Spinal manipulative therapy for low back pain. A metaanalysis of effectiveness relative to other therapies. Ann Intern Med 2003;138:871–81.
36. Cherkin DC, Sherman KJ, Deyo RA, et al. A review of the evidence for the effectiveness, safety, and cost of acupuncture, massage therapy, and spinal manipulation for back pain. Ann Intern Med 2003;138:898–906.
37. Haake M, Müller HH, Schade-Brittinger C, et al. German acupuncture trials (GERAC) for chronic low back pain. Arch Intern Med 2007;167(17):1892–8.
38. Manheimer E, White A, Berman B, et al. Meta-analysis: acupuncture for low back pain. Ann Intern Med 2005;142:651–63.
39. Brinkhaus B, Witt CM, Jena S, et al. Acupuncture in patients with chronic low back pain: a randomized controlled trial. Arch Intern Med 2006;166:450–7.
40. Cherkin DC, Sherman KJ, Avins AL, et al. A randomized trial comparing acupuncture, simulated acupuncture, and usual care for chronic low back pain. Arch Intern Med 2009;169(9):858–66.

41. French SD, Cameron M, Walker BF, et al. Superficial heat or cold for low back pain. Cochrane Database Syst Rev 2006;1:CD004750.
42. Cherkin DC, Eisenberg D, Sherman KJ, et al. Randomized trial comparing traditional Chinese medical acupuncture, therapeutic massage, and self-care education for chronic low back pain. Arch Intern Med 2001;161:1081–8.
43. Clarke JA, van Tulder MW, Blomberg SE, et al. Traction for low-back pain with or without sciatica. Cochrane Database Syst Rev 2005;4:CD003010.
44. Chou R, Huffman LH, for the American Pain Society and the American College of Physicians. Nonpharmacologic therapies for acute and chronic low back pain: a review of the evidence for an American Pain Society/American College of Physicians clinical practice guideline. Ann Intern Med 2007;147(7):492–504.
45. Frost H, Lamb SE, Doll HA, et al. Randomised controlled trial of physiotherapy compared with advice for low back pain. BMJ 2004;329:708.
46. Henrotin YE, Cedraschi C, Duplan B, et al. Information and low back pain management: a systematic review. Spine 2006;31:E326–34.
47. Damush TM, Weinberger M, Perkins SM, et al. The long-term effects of a self-management program for inner-city primary care patients with acute low back pain. Arch Intern Med 2003;163:2632–8.

Fibromyalgia: Helping Your Patient While Maintaining Your Sanity

Carol P. Motley, MD*, Meredith L. Maxwell, MD, MHA

KEYWORDS

• Fibromyalgia • Muscle pain • Joint pain • Tender points

Fibromyalgia has been known by many different names, including fibrositis, muscular rheumatism, and neurasthenia. It is a syndrome characterized by chronic widespread musculoskeletal pain and tenderness on specific areas of the body for at least 3 months.[1–3] Although the diagnosis and treatment of fibromyalgia may be daunting and somewhat confusing, in the last decade, pain research has led to a better understanding of fibromyalgia as a chronic pain state with disordered sensory processing and a diversity of clinical presentations.[1]

The American College of Rheumatology (ACR) published criteria for fibromyalgia in 1990, recognizing fibromyalgia as a chronic, painful, noninflammatory syndrome involving muscles rather than joints.[4–6] A range of symptoms could now be diagnosed as fibromyalgia and be distinguished from similar disorders.

Fibromyalgia is defined by the ACR as chronic (>3 months), widespread pain (axial plus upper and lower segment plus left- and right-sided pain), and tenderness in at least 11 of 18 anatomic points.[7]

INCIDENCE AND EPIDIMEOLOGY

Nearly 2% of the United States population is affected by fibromyalgia.[8,9] It is approximately 6 times more common in women (3.4%) than in men (0.5%).[10–12] It can occur in any age group, but women 20 to 50 years old are more likely to be affected.[10] Prevalence seems to increase with age, from 2% at age 20 years to 8% at age 70 years.[11,13]

The cost of fibromyalgia is high. In multiple studies, work loss in patients with fibromyalgia showed 20% to 50% of subjects with no or few days lost, 36% with 2 or more

Financial Support: None

Department of Family Medicine, University of South Alabama, 1504 Springhill Avenue, Suite 3414, Mobile, AL 36604, USA

* Corresponding author.

E-mail address: cmotley@usouthal.edu

Prim Care Clin Office Pract 37 (2010) 743–755

doi:10.1016/j.pop.2010.07.007

days lost per month, and 26.5% to 55% who collected disability or social security and did not work at all.[14–16]

PATHOPHYSIOLOGY

Any discussion of pathophysiology must begin with questions of the existence of fibromyalgia as a distinct clinical entity. Evidence against the existence of fibromyalgia includes a lack of a clear cause and treatment, the absence of specific abnormalities, and the difficulties in assessment of the physical complaints of disability made by patients with fibromyalgia.[13] Others attribute the pain, fatigue, and cognitive dysfunction to depression, an inappropriate response to stress, or a somatoform disorder.[13] Investigators who supported this belief concluded that it would then be a learned pattern of maladaptive behavior and not a distinctive disorder.[3]

There are clear data supporting fibromyalgia as a distinct clinical syndrome. There is ample evidence from physiologic and genetic investigations that changes have occurred in patients with fibromyalgia, but causation has not been established. There is a connection between neurobiological, psychosocial, and behavioral factors, and patients with fibromyalgia are no different.[5] There are characteristic changes in sleep patterns and alterations in neuroendocrine transmitters suggesting that dysregulation of the autonomic and neuroendocrine system is the basis of the syndrome. The evidence for a physiologic basis for the illness is presented in **Table 1**.[12,14] In addition, there is some overlap with certain metabolic disorders. Fibromyalgia is more prevalent in women with thyroid disease and in men and women infected with human immunodeficiency virus.[13] Women with hyperprolactinemia develop fibromyalgia at a rate 15 times that of their nonaffected peers.[13] Reports of antecedent infections with hepatitis C, Epstein-Barr virus, parvovirus, and Lyme disease exist but causality has not been established.[5,15]

PRESENTING SYMPTOMS

Pain is the major symptom of fibromyalgia and has been described as burning, stiffness, contracture, and tension.[17] Stiffness tends to be worse in the morning and decreases throughout the day.[10] The pain is chronic and persistent in nature with varying intensities and manifests itself throughout the body. It may originate from 1 localized point, such as the neck, spine, or shoulders, and move to other points such as the back, chest, hips, arms, and legs with time.[2,17] Tender points are generally positioned over muscles or sites where muscles insert. Two important features are a subjective feeling of a swollen joint or limb without objective swelling, and paresthesias without objective neurologic findings.[10]

Fatigue is present in more than 90% of cases of fibromyalgia and is occasionally the chief complaint.[11,13] Patients complain of feeling exhausted, even on waking. If fatigue is not present, the diagnosis should be held in question.

Headaches are reported by almost 75% of patients with fibromyalgia, the most common type of headache being migraine.[18] Depression is found in approximately half of patients afflicted with fibromyalgia, as is spastic colon and chronic fatigue in 70% of patients.[17] Also suggestive of fibromyalgia are a history of environmental sensitivities and restless leg syndrome.

Fibromyalgia symptoms vary in relation with the time of day, the level of activity, weather conditions (specifically cold and humid weather), and levels of sleep and stress.[10,17] Symptoms seem to be improved by warm and dry weather, moderate physical activity, adequate sleep, and relaxation.[10]

Table 1 Evidence for physiologic basis for fibromyalgia		
System	Evidence Supporting Distinct Pathologic Syndrome	Evidence Against Distinct Pathologic Syndrome
Pain perception	• Lower threshold for nociceptive processing • Persistent excitability of dorsal horn neurons • Altered levels of proprioceptive and antinociceptive compounds • Altered endogenous analgesia system, formerly innocuous stimuli now noxious	
Musculoskeletal		• No differences between patients with fibromyalgia and sedentary controls in terms of ATP levels, lactate levels, muscle tension, hypoxia, or intracellular pH on biopsy
Neuroendocrine	• Increased substance P • Decreased serotonin • Increased cortisol with flattened diurnal pattern • Disrupted dopamine release • Decreased growth hormone production	• Some patients show no altered cortisol response
Sleep disturbance	• Almost all have α-δ sleep anomaly with disrupted stage 4 sleep • Longer to initiate sleep • Repeated awakenings	
Genetics	• Increased incidence in first-degree relatives	
Environmental triggers	• Half of all cases have distinct physical or emotional trigger • Gulf War veterans have increased incidence	

Data from Desmules J, Cedraschi C, Rapiti E. Neurophysiologic evidence for a central sensitization in patients with fibromyalgia. Arthritis Rheum 2003;48:1420–7; and Staud R. Evidence of involvement of central neural mechanisms in generating fibromyalgia pain. Curr Rheum Rep 2002;4:299–305.

RISK FACTORS

Certain life stressors increase the risk of fibromyalgia. These include being divorced, failing to complete high school, and having a lower income.[10,13,17] In addition, other factors associated with fibromyalgia include the presence of somatization disorder, anxiety disorder, increased global severity of psychiatric illness, history of abuse, history of past or current depression, and family history of depression.[13,19]

DIAGNOSIS

A comprehensive history and physical are necessary to make an accurate diagnosis of fibromyalgia,[5] with particular attention to sleep/fatigue, pain, mood, and exercise or work intolerance.[12] The fibromyalgia profile includes widespread pain, hypersensitivity at palpation in specific anatomic points, accompanied by the multisystem features of fibromyalgia, especially constant fatigue, sleep problems, and paresthesias.[8,12] Pain in all 4 body quadrants for at least 3 months should lead a provider to investigate for the presence of tender points, assess for pain, and entertain the diagnosis of fibromyalgia.[12]

The diagnosis is made if a patient has a 3-month history of widespread pain with the presence of 11 tender points among 18 specific anatomic sites.[10,20] Axial pain should be a constant attribute, and that pain must be present in both the upper and lower quadrants and the right and left sides of the body,[12] and tender points have specific anatomic sites bilaterally (**Fig. 1**).[10,12] The clinician must methodically palpate the

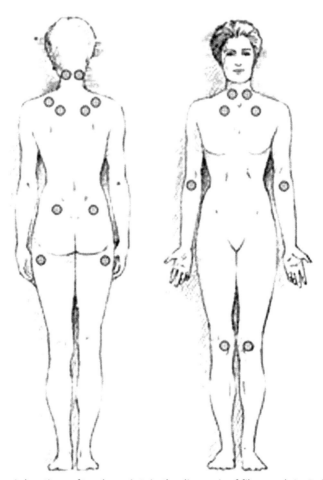

Fig. 1. Anatomic locations of tender points in the diagnosis of fibromyalgia. Definitive diagnosis requires 3 months of pain and the presence of tenderness in 11 of 18 sites. (*From* Freundlich B, Leventhal L. The Fibromyalgia syndrome. In: Schumacher HR, Klippel JH, Koopman WJ, editors. Primer on the Rheumatic diseases. 10th edition. Atlanta (GA): Arthritis Foundation; 1993; with permission.)

18 sites with steady pressure using the thumb of the dominant hand.[5,10] The pressure should be enough to turn the thumbnail white.[5] Tender points lack the classic signs of inflammation such as erythema, edema, and warmth in joints and soft tissue.[5,12] It is common for the most significant areas of pain to shift over time and the number of tender points to change over time.[12] These criteria provide a sensitivity and specificity of nearly 85% in differentiating fibromyalgia from other forms of chronic musculoskeletal pain.[20] Failure to meet these criteria does not absolutely exclude the possibility of fibromyalgia.

There are no confirmatory laboratory tests. Limited laboratory testing should be used to broaden the differential diagnosis. Tests should include a complete blood count, erythrocyte sedimentation rate, tests of thyroid function, hepatitis C antibodies, and creatinine phosphokinase.[5,21] Further testing should be based on clinical indications.[10] As with other rheumatologic disorders, symptoms exist on a continuum and the diagnosis is best established with observation over time.[12] The time between onset of fibromyalgia until diagnosis and treatment typically ranges from months to years.

DIFFERENTIAL DIAGNOSIS

Fibromyalgia symptoms may mimic many other diseases such as rheumatoid arthritis, hypothyroidism, sleep apnea, depression, and vitamin D deficiency.[8] Additional possibilities include mononucleosis, diabetes mellitus, multiple sclerosis, Sjogren disease, and Lyme disease.[5]

Diagnostic criteria of chronic fatigue syndrome (CFS) are similar to those for fibromyalgia, and most patients with CFS meet tender point criteria for fibromyalgia. Similarly, about 70% of patients with fibromyalgia meet the criteria for CFS.[12] However, patients with CFS typically have continuous subclinical inflammatory process and associated low-grade fever, lymph gland enlargement, and acute onset of illness.[12]

Confusion between fibromyalgia and polymyalgica rheumatica (PMR) often occurs with elderly patients.[8] PMR is characterized by stiffness in the sacrohumeral and pelvic girdle.[17] The erythrocyte sedimentation rate is increased in 80% to 90% of patients with PMR, and symptoms disappear with the use of corticosteroids, neither of which is seen in fibromyalgia.[12,17] The diagnosis for PMR, CFS, myofascial syndrome, and fibromyalgia often overlap and care should be taken to assign the correct diagnosis. These similarities and differences are summarized in **Table 2**.

Other diagnoses include drug-induced myopathies seen with colchicine, statins, corticosteroids, or antimalarials. In addition, connective tissue, autoimmune, and rheumatologic disorders such as spondyloarthropathy, dermatomyositis, and systemic lupus erythematosis can present in this manner but can usually be distinguished from fibromyalgia based on clinical criteria.[5,12] The characteristic synovitis and systemic features of connective tissue disorders are usually not features of fibromyalgia.[12] In the absence of findings characteristic of these illnesses, routine serologic testing should not be performed.

TREATMENT

Current treatment goals for patients with fibromyalgia are focused on symptom relief. Generally, this includes controlling pain, increasing restorative sleep, and improving physical function, well-being, and adjustment.[5]

Table 2
Similarities and differences between fibromyalgia, CFS, polymyalgia rheumatica, and myofascial syndrome

Disorder	Diagnostic Criteria	Inflammatory Signs	Sedimentation Rate
Fibromyalgia	Local tenderness, occurring in multiple specific locations that do not cause referred pain, but often cause a total body increase in pain sensitivity	Pain may get worse in response to activity, stress, weather changes	Normal ESR
Polymyalgia rheumatica	≥3 of the following, or ≥1 of the following plus positive results on temporal artery biopsy: • Bilateral shoulder pain and/or stiffness • <2 weeks from onset of symptoms to maximal symptoms • ESR>40 mm/h • Morning stiffness >1 h • Patient>65 y • Depression and/or weight loss • Bilateral upper arm tenderness	Pain and stiffness in shoulder and pelvic girdle greatest in morning and lasting 30–60 min after patients arises	Increased ESR
Chronic fatigue syndrome	≥4 of following symptoms for ≥6 mo: • Impaired memory or concentration • Postexertional malaise • Unrefreshing sleep • Muscle pain • Multijoint pain without swelling or redness • Headaches of new type or severity • Frequent or recurring sore throat • Tender cervical or axillary nodes	Myalgias, arthralgias, sore throat, lymphadenopathy, headaches	Normal ESR
Myofascial pain syndrome	Local tenderness, taut band trigger points, singular or multiple, may occur in any skeletal muscle, may cause a specific referred pain pattern	Regional, persistent pain (especially of postural muscles) that usually results in decreased range of motion of muscle in question	Normal ESR

Abbreviation: ESR, erythrocyte sedimentation rate.
From Martinez-Lanvin M. Overlap of fibromyalgia with other medical condtions. Curr Pain Headache Rep 2001;5:247–50; and *from* Freundlick B, Leventhal L. The fibromyalgia syndrome. In: Schumacher HR, Kilippel JH, Koopman WJ, editors. Primer on the rheumatic diseases. 10th edition. Atlanta (GA): Arthritis Foundation; 1993. p. 428–40.

Pharmacologic

Antidepressants

There is good evidence supporting the use of antidepressants in the treatment of patients with fibromyalgia to reduce symptoms.[10,11] In 2004, the American Pain Society issued fibromyalgia treatment recommendations that include tricyclic antidepressants (TCAs), selective serotonin reuptake inhibitors (SSRIs), and tramadol.[3,22] Updated guidelines suggest the use of serotonin-norepinephrine reuptake inhibitors (SNRIs), such as venlafaxine or duloxetine, and also recommend gabapentin or pregabalin (Lyrica).[3] Similarly, the United States Food and Drug Administration (FDA) has approved tricyclics, SNRIs, and pregabalin.[12] Most of the evidence for efficacy has been developed using amitriptyline and the muscle relaxant cyclobenzaprine (structurally similar to the TCAs), but there is no evidence of superiority of one class of antidepressants over another.[15,20]

TCAs

TCAs act by increasing serotonin and norepinephrine.[15] The efficacy of the tricyclic, amitriptyline, in fibromyalgia has been well documented.[4,20,22] Low dosages of 25 to 50 mg at bedtime, provide an analgesic effect and improve sleep and mood disorders.[10] Approximately one-third of patients with fibromyalgia show moderate short-term improvements in pain, disturbed sleep, patient and physician global assessments, physical status, psychological status, and capacity for activities of daily living with amitriptyline.[12]

Anticholinergic and sedative side effects of TCAs are the limiting factor in treating some patients. Tolerance can be improved by starting low (5–10 mg) and titrating up slowly (5-mg increase every 2 weeks), with the final dose set by the patient based on efficacy and side effects.[12,15] Desipramine (Norpramin) is less studied than amitriptyline, but has fewer anticholinergic side effects and may be a reasonable alternative.[12] A tricyclic should be used at least 6 weeks before a trial is considered unsuccessful.[5]

Cyclobenzaprine (Flexeril)

Although usually marketed as a muscle relaxant, cyclobenzaprine is structurally a tricyclic compound.[20] The benefits of treatment typically substantially outweigh the potential risks and clinicians should discuss the use of this medication with eligible patients. Evidence suggests using cyclobenzaprine at 10 to 30 mg at bedtime improves sleep quality and pain symptoms for patients with fibromyalgia.[2,4,10,20]

SSRIs

This class of antidepressants can help relieve pain and depression for patients with fibromyalgia and may be better tolerated than tricyclics.[2,23] One study found that increasing doses of paroxetine (Paxil) significantly improved the overall symptoms of fibromyalgia.[2,23] The trial used the Fibromyalgia Impact Questionnaire (FIQ) to measure symptoms. Items on the FIQ measure work status, depression, anxiety, morning tiredness, pain, stiffness, fatigue, and well-being.[4,10,20,24]

Studies have found greater improvement when TCAs and SSRIs are used together. Fluoxetine (Prozac) 20 mg/d and amitriptyline 25 mg/d were more effective when administered together than when administered separately.[23] As with other patients, there may be an increased suicidal tendency associated with SSRIs, and these patients should be monitored accordingly.[12]

SNRIs

Although similar to tricyclics, the SNRIs exhibit fewer side effects. The doses needed for fibromyalgia are generally higher than those required to treat depression.[12]

Venlafaxine (Effexor) increases serotonin at low doses and norepinephrine at higher doses (typically at doses of more than 100 mg).[12] Another SNRI, milnacipran (Savella), lacks anticholinergic, antihistaminic and α-adrenergic receptor blockade, improving the side effect profile.[6] Milnacipran exhibits a threefold greater efficacy in inhibiting norepinephrine reuptake compared with serotonin reuptake (in vitro), seems to be safe and well tolerated, and has shown a modest improvement in symptoms of fibromyalgia (pain, global impressions of change, and physical functioning).[20,25]

Duloxetine (Cymbalta), a potent SNRI with virtually no cholinergic, histaminic, or adrenergic activity, is approved by the FDA for the treatment of fibromyalgia, depression and diabetic neuropathy.[12] Relief of pain and tenderness was demonstrated with a dose of 60 mg twice daily.[10,12]

Anticonvulsant drugs

Antiseizure medications have shown efficacy in neuropathic pain syndromes and are often used as analgesics. Although their anticonvulsant activity occurs through slowing electrical signals in the brain, these drugs also subdue the transmission of pain signals.[12] Pregabalin (Lyrica), 450 mg/d, shows benefit in diffuse pain, sleep disturbances, and fatigue associated with fibromyalgia,[8] and has been shown to significantly reduced the average severity of fibromyalgia pain (up to 50%) compared with placebo.[10,15] Improvements in sleep, fatigue, and health-related quality of life were also seen among those receiving 300 and 400 mg/d.[15]

Analgesics

Tramadol has shown benefit in fibromyalgia pain.[1,10,20] Effectiveness of tramadol may be to the result of its weak μ-agonist activity combined with serotonin-norepinephrine reuptake inhibition.[15] Tramadol at 200 to 300 mg/d has a modest efficacy in treating fibromyalgia.[20] Because there is no inflammatory process found in fibromyalgia, nonsteroidal antiinflammatory drugs (NSAIDs) alone have not been effective.[10,12] Therapeutic doses of naproxen, ibuprofen, and prednisone (20 mg/d) were found to be no better than placebo in clinical trials.[12] However, NSAIDs may have a synergistic effect when combined with medications such as antidepressants or anticonvulsants.[12]

Sedative hypnotics

Benzodiazepines and sedatives have proven ineffective.[12] Nonbenzodiazepine hypnotics, such as zopiclone and zolpidem, can improve sleep patterns and fatigue of patients with fibromyalgia, but there has been no significant improvement on pain modulation.[15]

Opioid analgesia

Because of the augmented central pain processing, opioid medications, which are commonly used to treat peripheral pain, are not as effective in fibromyalgia.[12] The use of opioids has been associated with worsening of certain types of chronic pain.[26] Pharmacologic agents that downregulate central sensory processing are preferred for disease states such as fibromyalgia.[15] Many patients were started on long-term narcotic therapy before pharmacologic agents that improved central pain syndrome were available. These patients need to have medications added to treat the central pain syndrome with the goal of reducing or eliminating the use of narcotic analgesia.

Even with the newer medication, there are patients in whom the use of long-term opioid therapy cannot be avoided. Although beyond the scope of this discussion, these medications should only be initiated in consultation with a specialist in the field.

The patient should be made aware that long-term use of moderate to high opioid doses will likely result in physical dependence. In addition, tolerance typically develops, necessitating increasing dosages over time. For these patients, a multidisciplinary team approach should be used.

Other
The efficacy of human growth hormone was studied in a small trial that showed significant improvement compared with placebo, but the benefit was lost when the therapy was stopped. The costs of such treatment were considered to be excessive and further investigation was not pursued.[27] One small study demonstrated improvement in patients with a borderline high erythrocyte sedimentation rate (ESR) using low-dose naltrexone. There is a more extensive trial underway at this time.[28]

Nonpharmacologic

Guidelines from the American Pain Society recommend cognitive behavioral therapy (CBT) and moderate aerobic and muscle strengthening exercises in the treatment of fibromyalgia.[22] Other nonpharmacologic strategies include mind-body cognitive therapy, and complementary and alternative therapies.

Exercise
Supervised aerobic exercise training has beneficial effects on increasing physical capacity and decreasing fibromyalgia symptoms.[4,10] Reduction of pain was the primary benefit seen in patients who participated in an structured exercise program that included strength, aerobic conditioning, flexibility, and balance,[10] which are dimensions that should be included in any exercise program. The exercise program should be low impact and of sufficient intensity to change aerobic capacity. In addition, improvement in mood and physical function was documented.[29] In a 2009 Cochrane Review of a moderate-intensity aerobic training for 12 weeks, including cardiorespiratory endurance, muscle strengthening, and/or flexibility using the American College of Sports Medicine guidelines, found benefits in global outcome measures, physical function, and possibly pain and tender points.[14,30] Strength training can also reduce pain, tender points, and depression in patients with fibromyalgia.[10,14,30]

Patients should start slow and exercise at their own pace because exacerbation of pain may reduce compliance.[12] If exercisers experience increased symptoms, they should cut back until symptoms improve, although no serious side effects of exercise have been documented.[14,30] A controlled exercise program may ameliorate the cycle of pain that perpetuates a lack of physical activity, related depression, and more pain.[14,31] Better muscular blood flow, less susceptibility to muscular microtrauma, and an improvement in sleep as a result of regular training contribute to improved symptoms.[14,31] The type and intensity of exercise should be patient specific according to abilities, preferences, and goals.[2,14,32] For example, water exercise has been well tolerated and is especially helpful because these exercises are low impact and warm water may help reduce stiffness and pain.[2,20] Although the benefit of exercise persisted even after cessation, ongoing exercise is recommended for sustained benefit.[20,33] The type and intensity of exercise should be patient specific according to abilities, preferences, and goals.[2,14,32,34] In Germany, continuous pool- and land-based exercises and support groups are reimbursed by health insurance companies.[7]

CBT
CBT teaches patients to understand the effects that negative thoughts, beliefs, and expectations have on their symptoms.[10,35] Patients often have counterproductive

ways of thinking and acting that only make their symptoms worse.[35] CBT should be considered as an adjunctive therapy in the management of patients with fibromyalgia, particularly those who present with an emotionally distressed and/or dysfunctional profile.[35] The rationale for use of CBT in the management of patients with fibromyalgia is based, in part, on the physiologic links between chronic pain and depression.[35] CBT can help teach patients how to manage anger, stress, and anxieties that may be contributing to, and may result from, fibromyalgia symptoms.[35] Patients can learn how to "adapt daily activities to prevent flare-ups caused by doing too much or lethargy caused by doing too little."[2]

CBT has been shown in small trials to positively affect pain severity, life interference, sense of control, affective distress, depression, perceived physical impairment, fatigue, and anxiety.[15,20,35] The benefit of CBT can be achieved in 10 to 20 sessions.[35]

Patient education and self-efficacy

A diagnosis of fibromyalgia may lead to increasing disability and can facilitate a state of learned helplessness, or it can be a turning point, allowing the patient to focus on managing the syndrome.[2] Evidence is limited, but patients who have been diagnosed have significant improvements in health satisfaction and symptoms, and use fewer health resources.[12] The diagnosis of fibromyalgia should be coupled with patient education, which may be as effective as CBT.[32] High self-efficacy (patient's sense of personal control in the management of their symptoms) before beginning an exercise program predicts positive changes in disease severity, increased physical activity, and better pain outcomes.[32,36,37] The goal of education should be to shift the patient's perception from one of helplessness, frustration, and sometimes anger to a positive sense of self-efficacy and hope.[32] The Arthritis Self-help Course has been highly successful in changing patient self-efficacy and health behavior, and in reducing physician visits and health care costs.[32] A fibromyalgia -specific self-help course is now available through the Arthritis Foundation at www.arthritis.org.

The severity of fibromyalgia symptoms seems to correlate with less deep restorative sleep.[12] Sleep quality seems to be an indicator for controlling the symptoms of fibromyalgia, especially muscle pain and fatigue symptoms. Circumstances interfering with stage 4 deep sleep (such as drug use, pain, or anxiety) seem to worsen the symptoms associated with fibromyalgia.[24] Good sleep quality may moderate the relationship between affect and pain such that a good night's sleep increases the ability to resist bouts of pain; alternatively, poor sleep, especially when chronic, may increase vulnerability to fibromyalgia symptoms.[24]

Alternative therapies

There is limited evidence for the effectiveness of alternative therapies. These therapies are summarized in **Table 3**.

Multicomponent treatment

The doctor-patient relationship is important. The degree of patient satisfaction at the conclusion of a physician-patient encounter is a significant determinant of overall patient compliance.[12] The generally accepted approach to treating fibromyalgia is a multimodal regimen that includes patient education, CBT, gentle exercise, and medications to help with sleep and pain.[1,20] Multidisciplinary rehabilitation is typically included despite a Cochrane Review conclusion that there seems to be little scientific evidence for the effectiveness. Combining education, CBT, or both with exercise produces beneficial effects on patient self-efficacy, pain, and on 6-minute walk testing.[20,32]

Table 3 Alternative therapies in fibromyalgia	
Alternative Therapy	**Proposed Benefits**
Stress reduction via meditation	Eases pain, improves sleep and concentration, alleviates depression
Acupuncture	Increased pain thresholds Decreased pain ratings
Hypnotherapy	Eases pain, improves sleep and concentration, alleviates depression
Biofeedback	Reduced pain ratings
Balneotherapy	Increased pain thresholds Decreased pain ratings
Transcranial direct current stimulation	Decreased pain ratings

Data from Berman B, Ezzo J, Hadhazy V, et al. Is acupuncture effective in the treatment of fibromyalgia? J Fam Pract 1999;48:213–8; and Crofford L, Appleton B. Complementary and alternative therapies for fibromyalgia. Curr Rheum Rep 2001;3:147–56.

PROGNOSIS

Most patients with fibromyalgia continue to have chronic pain and fatigue. Despite little change in symptoms in 14 years, two-thirds of patients reported that they were working full time and that fibromyalgia interfered only modestly with their lives.[12] If the patient has a sense of control over pain, a belief that he or she is not disabled, and understands that pain is not a sign of damage, the prognosis is better.[12] Other behaviors associated with better outcomes included seeking help from others, decreasing guarding during examination, exercising more, and pacing activities.[12]

MANAGEMENT STRATEGY

A stepwise approach to fibromyalgia management has been suggested. First, confirm the diagnosis, explain the condition, and evaluate and treat comorbid illness. Second, begin a trial with low-dose TCAs or cyclobenzaprine. Instruct the patient on how to begin a cardiovascular fitness exercise program. Then, refer for CBT or stress reduction with relaxation training. Lastly, consider trying an SSRI, SNRI, or tramadol. Also consider a combination medication trial or anticonvulsant. If the patient is not responding well to these steps, refer to a rheumatologist, physiatrist, psychiatrist, or pain management specialist.[20]

SUMMARY

The primary care provider plays an important role in the diagnosis and treatment of patients with fibromyalgia. The clinician should have a low index of suspicion for the syndrome in patients who have complaints of myalgias and fatigue. There is no single, effective treatment of fibromyalgia. Pharmacologic and nonpharmacologic treatment must be individualized to each patient, and a trial of a variety of different therapeutic methods may be necessary. Ideally, the practitioner will collaborate with the patient to construct a unique treatment plan for the patient's circumstances that includes a team-based approach.

REFERENCES

1. Bennett R, Kamin M, Karim R, et al. Tramadol and acetaminophen combination tablets in the treatment of fibromyalgia pain: a double-blind, randomized, placebo-controlled study. Am J Med 2003;114:537–45.
2. The best way to treat fibromyalgia. It may require more than one strategy, but you can get some pain relief and feel a lot better about life. Harv Women's Health Watch 2004;11:4–5.
3. White L, Robinson R, Yu A, et al. Comparison of health care use and costs in newly diagnosed and established patients with fibromyalgia. J Pain 2009;10(9): 976–83.
4. Dadabhoy D, Crofford L, Spaeth M, et al. Biology and therapy of fibromyalgia. Evidence-based biomarkers for fibromyalgia syndrome. Arthritis Res Ther 2008;10:211.
5. Peterson E. Fibromyalgia - management of a misunderstood disorder. J Am Acad Nurse Pract 2007;19:241–348.
6. WolfeSmythe H, Yanus M. The American College of Rheumatology criteria for the classification of fibromyalgia. Report of the Multicenter Criteria Committee. Arthritis Rheum 1990;33:160–72.
7. Hauser W, Bernardy K, Arnold B, et al. Efficacy of multicomponent treatment in fibromyalgia syndrome: a meta-analysis of randomized controlled clinical trials. Arthritis Rheum 2009;61(2):216–24.
8. Martinez-Lanvin M. Overlap of fibromyalgia with other medical conditions. Curr Pain Headache Rep 2001;5:347–50.
9. Buskila D, Sarzi-Puttini P. Genetic aspects of fibromyalgia syndrome. Arthritis Res Ther 2006;8(218):1–5.
10. Chakkrabarty S, Zoorob R. Fibromyalgia. Am Fam Physician 2007;76(2):247–54.
11. O'Malley P, Balden E, Tomkins G, et al. Treatment of fibromyalgia with antidepressants: a meta-analysis. J Gen Intern Med 2000;15:659–66.
12. Millea P, Holloway R. Treating fibromyalgia. Am Fam Physician 2000. Available at: http://www.aafp.org/afp/AFPprinter/2000v1001/1575.html. Accessed March 9, 2009.
13. White K, Harth M. Classification, epidemiology, and natural history of fibromyalgia. Curr Pain Headache Rep 2001;5:320–9.
14. Busch AJ, Barber KA, Overend TJ, et al. Exercise for treating fibromyalgia syndrome. Cochrane Database Syst Rev 2007;4:CD003786.
15. Dadabhoy D, Clauw D. Therapy insight: fibromyalgia - a different type of pain needing a different type of treatment. Nat Clin Pract Rheumatol 2006;2(7):364–72.
16. Wolfe F, Anderson J, Harkness D, et al. Work and disability status of persons with fibromyalgia. J Rheumatol 1997;24(6):1171–8.
17. Coaccioli S, Varrassi G, Sabatini C, et al. Fibromyalgia: nosography and therapeutic perspectives. Pain Pract 2008;8:190–201.
18. Marcus D, Bernstein C, Rudy T. Fibromyalgia and headache: an epidemiological study supporting migraine as part of the fibromyalgia syndrome. Clin Rheumatol 2005;24:595–601.
19. Eisen S, Kang H, Murphy F, et al. Gulf war veterans' health: medical evaluation of a U.S. Cohort. Ann Intern Med 2005;142(11):881–90.
20. Goldenberg D, Burckhardt C, Crofford L. Management of fibromyalgia syndrome. JAMA 2004;292:2388–95.
21. Freundlich B, Leventhal L. The fibromyalgia syndrome. In: Schumacher HR, Klippel JH, Koopman WJ. Primer on the rheumatic diseases. 10th edition. Atlanta (GA): Arthritis Foundation; 1993. p. 428–40.

22. Buckhardt C, Goldenberg D, Crofford L, et al. Guidelines for the management of fibromyalgia syndrome pain in adults and children. Glenview (IL): American Pain Society (APS); 2005. (Clinical practice guideline; no. 4).

23. Arnold L, Haess E, Hudson J, et al. A randomized, placebo-controlled, double-blind, flexible-dose study of fluoxetine in the treatment of women with fibromyalgia. Am J Med 2002;112:191–7.

24. Bigatti S, Hernandez A, Cronan T, et al. Sleep disturbances in fibromyalgia syndrome: relationship to pain and depression. Arthritis Rheum 2008;59(7): 961–7.

25. Mease P, Clauw J, Gendreau, et al. The efficacy and safety of milnacipran for treatment of fibromyalgia. A randomized, double-blind, placebo controlled trial. J Rheumatol 2009;36(2):398–409.

26. Chu D, Clark D, Angst M. Opioid tolerance and hyperalgesia in chronic pain patients after one month of oral morphine therapy; a preliminary prospective study. J Pain 2006;7:43–8.

27. Bennett R, Clark S, Wlaczyk J. A randomized, double-blind, placebo-controlled study of growth hormone in the treatment of fibromyalgia. Am J Med 1998;20: 227–31.

28. Younger J, Mackey S. Low-dose naltrexone reduces the primary symptoms of fibromyalgia. Pain Med 2009;10(4):663–72.

29. Gowans S, deHueck A, Voss S, et al. Effect of a randomized, controlled trial of exercise on mood and physical function in individuals with fibromyalgia. Arthritis Rheum 2001;45:519–29.

30. Busch A, Barber K, Overend T, et al. Exercise for treating fibromyalgia syndrome. Cochrane Database Syst Rev 2007;4.

31. Meiworm L, Jakob E, Walker U, et al. Patients with fibromyalgia benefit from aerobic endurance exercise. Clin Rheumatol 2000;19:253–7.

32. Burckhardt C. Nonpharmacologic management strategies in fibromyalgia. Rheum Dis Clin North Am 2002;28:291–304.

33. Gowans S, deHueck A, Silaj A, et al. Six-month and one-year follow-up of 23 weeks of aerobic exercise for individuals with fibromyalgia. Arthritis Rheum 2004;51(6):890–8.

34. Berman B, Ezzo J, Hadhazy V, et al. Is acupuncture effective in the treatment of fibromyalgia? J Fam Pract 1999;48:213–8.

35. Bennett R, Nelson D. Cognitive behavioral therapy for fibromyalgia. Nat Clin Pract Rheumatol 2006;2(8):416–24.

36. Buckelew S, Parker J, Keefe F, et al. Self-efficacy and pain behavior among subjects with fibromyalgia. Pain 1994;59(3):377–84.

37. McCain G, Bell D, Mai F, et al. A controlled study of the effects of a supervised cardiovascular fitness training program on the manifestations of primary fibromyalgia. Arthritis Rheum 1988;31:1135–41.

Temporal Arteritis: An Approach to Suspected Vasculitides

Natasha Harder, MD[a,b]

KEYWORDS

- Temporal arteritis • Giant cell arteritis • Vasculitis
- Polymyalgia rheumatica • Monocular vision loss
- Headache • Jaw claudication • Diplopia

Temporal arteritis is a panarteritis that involves the extracranial branches of the carotid artery preferentially and is the most common vasculitis in adults.[1] The condition was first described by Hutchinson in 1890 and then was not discussed again until the 1930s when the histology of the granulomatous vessels was described.[2] Temporal arteritis can have a variable clinical presentation, which can range from chronic headache to monocular vision loss.[3] Because of the array of presenting complaints and the significant sequelae if untreated, primary care physicians need to be familiar with diagnosing and treating temporal arteritis.

EPIDEMIOLOGY

The incidence of temporal arteritis increases with age. The peak incidence is between 70 and 80 years of age, with a mean age of 72 years. It is rare for a person younger than 50 years to experience this disease.[4] The prevalence of temporal arteritis varies among different ethnic and racial groups. The disease occurs more often in whites than in blacks, Hispanics, or Asians. Geographically, prevalence increases from the southern to the northern latitudes.[5] Temporal arteritis is especially common in the people of the Scandinavian or the Northern European heritage.[1] Women are affected twice as often as men.[3]

Author has no financial conflicts of interest.
[a] Tuscaloosa Family Medicine Residency, University of Alabama School of Medicine, 850 5th Avenue East, Tuscaloosa, AL 35401, USA
[b] Department of Family Medicine, University of Alabama School of Medicine, 850 5th Avenue East Box 870377, Tuscaloosa, AL 35401, USA
E-mail address: nharder@cchs.ua.edu

Prim Care Clin Office Pract 37 (2010) 757–766
doi:10.1016/j.pop.2010.07.005
0095-4543/10/$ – see front matter © 2010 Published by Elsevier Inc.

primarycare.theclinics.com

PATHOGENESIS

The cause of temporal arteritis is not completely understood. One theory involves activation of the cellular immune response system involving T cells and macrophages,[2] which results in inflammatory changes to the arterial wall, causing intimal thickening and arterial narrowing. This narrowing of the artery can lead to thrombosis and possibly to the development of areas of ischemia or infarction.[6] As temporal arteritis most commonly affects branches of the internal and external carotid artery, the ischemia results in the symptoms of headache, jaw claudication, scalp tenderness, and blindness.[4] Granulomatous inflammation forms giant cells in the classic pathologic lesion and gives the disease its alternate name, giant cell arteritis.[3]

Infection has been suggested to play a role in the pathogenesis of temporal arteritis, with some studies noting an increase in the level of antibodies against several viruses and bacteria in these patients. These organisms may be the inciting cause of a cellular immune response that can cause the initial damage to the arterial wall. *Mycoplasma pneumoniae* and *Chlamydia pneumoniae* as well as parainfluenza virus, varicella-zoster virus, and parvovirus B19 have all been implicated as causative agents.[2] The cyclic nature of parvovirus B19, which fluctuates every 6 to 7 years, has been noted to coincide with similar fluctuations in the incidence of temporal arteritis. One study noted that parvovirus B19 DNA was detected by polymerase chain reaction analysis in the temporal artery biopsy tissue of patients with the disease. With more research, the relationship between parvovirus B19 and temporal arteritis can be better elucidated.[6]

CLINICAL PRESENTATION

There are several symptoms that are classically associated with the disease. The classic symptoms are polymyalgia rheumatica (PMR), headache, jaw claudication, and visual symptoms.[1] Although these are the classic symptoms, not every patient with temporal arteritis presents with these symptoms. There are multiple body systems that exhibit symptoms of this disease (**Table 1**).

PMR has been observed in 40% to 60% of patients with temporal arteritis, whereas approximately 10% of patients with PMR have concurrent temporal arteritis. PMR is characterized by severe pain and stiffness to the shoulder and pelvic girdle muscles or proximal muscle groups sparing the distal muscles. [2,4]

Headache is present in 70% of cases and is the most common clinical manifestation. The pain is usually centered over the temporal region but can occasionally be located over the occipital region as well. The most striking clinical feature of this headache is that it is new onset or characteristically different from previous headaches.[1]

Table 1 Symptoms of temporal arteritis	
Constitutional Symptoms	Fever, malaise, anorexia, weight loss[3]
Respiratory Symptoms	Dry cough, sore throat, hoarseness, sensation of choking[1]
Sensory Symptoms	Vision loss, amaurosis fugax, diplopia, hearing loss, vertigo[7,8]
Peripheral Nervous System	Mononeuropathies, polyneuropathies[5]
Central Nervous System	Headache, transient ischemic attack, central vascular accident, hallucination[1]
Musculoskeletal System	Jaw claudication, polymyalgia rheumatica, arthritis, tenosynovitis[1,2,9]
Cardiovascular System	Upper and lower extremity claudication, pitting edema[1]

A more specific complaint for temporal arteritis other than headache is scalp pain, which occurs in 40% of patients. A new-onset headache or scalp pain in patients older than 50 years should raise clinical suspicion of temporal arteritis.[7]

Jaw claudication or angina of the muscles of mastication is more often unilateral but can be bilateral. This symptom is the most specific historical clue for temporal arthritis.[1,5] Jaw claudication is most notable when the patient eats food that requires prolonged chewing or can be caused by prolonged singing or talking. The symptom may also present as tongue pain or chronic odynophagia. Necrotic lesions of the tongue progressing to complete necrosis within a few days are a rare but serious complication.[7]

Early suspicion and treatment of this disease in patients with transient visual symptoms can prevent progression to complete vision loss.[7] The inflammation inherent in temporal arteritis causes an anterior ischemic optic neuropathy, which can cause permanent vision loss.[3] Permanent vision loss is almost never the first symptom patients have of temporal arteritis and is rarely reversible with the treatment of the disease. Thus, early detection and treatment is important. Amaurosis fugax, described as a shade coming down over one eye, precedes blindness in 44% of patients. Diplopia and visual hallucinations are less common but may also precede vision loss.[3] Diplopia is caused by ischemia of lateral eye muscles. The condition is found in approximately 10% of patients and is a specific finding for temporal arteritis. Permanent vision loss occurs in approximately 15% of patients. Progression from transient vision loss to permanent vision loss occurs on average in 8.5 days.[7] This finding highlights the need for a high level of clinical suspicion and immediate diagnosis and treatment when the disease is present to preserve vision.

Multiple constitutional symptoms are also likely in temporal arteritis. These symptoms include fever, malaise, anorexia, and weight loss, which can be present in half of all patients.[3] Temporal arteritis is one of the findings in patients investigated for fever of unknown origin (FUO) and should be considered in the workup of FUO in those older than 50 years. Several FUO studies have revealed that temporal arteritis is responsible for 25% to 36% of FUO cases in older persons.[10]

Temporal arteritis is a vasculitis that affects medium to large arteries not only mainly in the head and neck but also anywhere in the body. Patients can manifest symptoms of this vasculitis as respiratory, peripheral nervous system, and central nervous system symptoms. One series estimated that 4% of patients have respiratory symptoms as the initial symptoms and 9% have respiratory symptoms as part of the total disease complex. The association of respiratory tract symptoms with the onset of temporal arteritis and their prompt alleviation with steroid therapy as well as their recurrence as the disease has relapses or exacerbations are all strong evidence that indicates that arteritis is the underlying cause.[11] Dry cough is the most common respiratory symptom. Other symptoms include sore throat, hoarseness, and the sensation of choking.[1] Ischemia in the affected tissues or a response to the inflammation of the arteries supplying these tissues is a likely explanation for these symptoms.[11] Involvement of the arteries that supply the otic region can lead to tinnitus, hearing loss, and vertigo.[8] Peripheral nervous system features include mononeuropathies and polyneuropathies.[5] Central nervous system manifestations include transient ischemic attacks, cerebral vascular accidents (CVAs), and hallucinations.[1] CVAs likely occur from vasculitis, thrombosis, and emboli formation from lesions in the internal carotid and vertebral arteries.[7]

Musculoskeletal manifestations can be more varied than just PMR. Arthritis was the most common peripheral manifestation, and bilateral symmetric involvement occurred in half of these episodes. These manifestations were of limited duration and responded to the initiation of steroids or an increase in the dosage if the patient was already taking steroids. This response was rapid and complete in most cases. Follow-up studies of these patients after resolution of temporal arteritis revealed that the arthritis resolved fully without residual joint changes. Distal extremity swelling with pitting edema, diffuse swelling without edema, and tenosynovitis can all be present in temporal arteritis. Studies of patients with these conditions have shown that these features are all variations of the same process, with the severity of tenosynovitis defining the clinical findings. Some patients have more extensive tenosynovitis with diffuse swelling and occasionally pitting edema, whereas others have a more localized inflammatory process and develop swelling that remains confined to the course of a specific tendon. Carpal tunnel syndrome that develops in patients who are currently being treated for temporal arteritis is most probably a tenosynovitis of the flexor tendons of the wrist.[9]

In approximately 10% to 15% of patients, the branches of the aortic arch, especially the subclavian and axillary arteries, become narrowed, which results in claudication of the upper extremities. Pulses in the neck or upper extremities may be decreased or absent, and blood pressures may be unequal in the upper extremities. Bruits may also be heard on auscultation over the carotid, subclavian, axillary, and brachial arteries. Lower extremity involvement that is extensive enough to cause claudication is rare but has been documented. The best diagnostic tests for detecting these extracranial manifestations of temporal arteritis are arteriography, computed tomography (CT), and magnetic resonance angiography. On arteriography, a smooth taped appearance is seen in the stenosis or occlusion of subclavian, axillary brachial, or femoral arteries.[1,2]

PHYSICAL EXAMINATION

On palpation, the temporal artery may be thickened, nodular, tender, or erythematous and the pulses decreased. An abnormal temporal artery is found on physical examination in only 50% of patients, so normal physical findings on palpation of the temporal artery do not rule out a diagnosis of temporal arteritis.[1,2]

The eye examination should assess vision and pupils for an afferent papillary defect, and a fundoscopic examination should evaluate the retina and optic disks. In those with vision loss from temporal arteritis, the fundoscopic examination shows pallor and edema of the optic disk, with scattered cotton-wool patches and small hemorrhages.[3]

DIAGNOSTIC TESTING

Diagnostic testing can include blood work and, in some centers, ultrasonography to assess the temporal artery. The gold standard test is the biopsy of the temporal artery. If clinical and laboratory findings suggest temporal arteritis, then biopsy should be performed by a surgeon sooner rather than later to confirm the diagnosis.[5]

Laboratory evaluation of temporal arteritis begins with the determination of the erythrocyte sedimentation rate (ESR). Most patients with temporal arteritis have an ESR of greater than 50 mm/h. There has been no normal ESR level established for temporal arteritis, but studies have suggested the use of the value of age/2 for men and (age + 10)/2 for women. Hence, there is a chance for wide variations of the ESR in temporal arteritis. Studies have documented levels of greater than 100 mm/h, and in one study, approximately 20% of patients had a normal ESR before treatment.[2] ESR is a nonspecific marker of inflammation, and an ESR value of greater than 50 mm/h has a reported specificity of 48% for temporal arteritis.[7]

C-reactive protein (CRP) is another marker of inflammation that can be used in the evaluation of temporal arteritis. Elevations of the levels of CRP greater than 6 mg/L have been reported in the literature. There have been conflicting reports on the accuracy of CRP and ESR usefulness for diagnosis. Using CRP and ESR together to increase the diagnostic yield is being investigated.[7]

Complete blood count typically shows a normocytic normochromic anemia and reactive thrombocytosis. Iron studies show findings consistent with anemia of chronic disease. These findings include low levels of serum iron, normal or elevated levels of ferritin, reduced levels of transferrin, and reduced total iron-binding capacity. Liver function tests frequently show elevated alkaline phosphatase levels, whereas elevation of the aspartate aminotransferase levels is seen less often.[8] Microscopic hematuria can be found on urinalysis in one-third of the patients.[7]

Color duplex ultrasonography is being investigated as a noninvasive means to investigate the temporal artery. Abnormal findings suggestive of temporal arteritis include a hyperechoic halo around the perfused lumen of the inflamed artery, stenosis of the artery, or complete occlusion.[12] If this technique is used, it should only be done by ultrasonographers who are trained to assess the temporal artery using specific protocols. In patients with temporal arteritis, the sensitivity and specificity of the diagnosis when confirmed by histology has been reported as 95% and 76%, respectively, when the characteristic abnormalities were observed.[13] In some centers, color duplex ultrasonography is being investigated as a diagnostic tool for temporal arteritis in patients with typical clinical and laboratory findings. Those patients who show a clear hyperechoic halo on ultrasonography are being considered for treatment without biopsy, unless other vasculitic syndromes are suspected. If the ultrasonography is normal or only occlusion or stenosis is seen, then a biopsy is recommended.[12] However, these recommendations are controversial because color duplex ultrasonography may not be able to distinguish between inflammatory and degenerative arterial disease.[14] Thus, the issue of color duplex ultrasonography requires more study before concrete recommendations can be made. If ultrasonography is used for diagnosis, it should be done by those who are skilled in imaging the temporal artery using protocols that have been proven. Until there is evidence otherwise, there should be no changes in the recommendations for biopsy to diagnose the disease.

The gold standard for the diagnosis of temporal arteritis is the temporal artery biopsy performed by a surgeon who is trained in this procedure. The amount of tissue needed varies based on the clinical findings. If there are localizing signs of temporal arteritis, such as tenderness or nodularity, then only a short segment needs to be biopsied. If, on the other hand, no tenderness or other signs of arteritis are present, a longer segment (3–5 cm) should be biopsied. Skip lesions are common in temporal arteritis, so the longer biopsy segment can help prevent missing the affected segment.[8] The issue of unilateral versus bilateral biopsy for the most accurate diagnosis is controversial. Recently 2 studies found that only 1% of patients with negative results on unilateral biopsy had positive results on contralateral biopsy. Other studies have found this number to be up to 3%. Because of the uncertainty, most surgeons continue to do a unilateral biopsy and only biopsy the contralateral side if the result of the first biopsy is negative on frozen section.[7] Treatment of temporal arteritis should not be delayed to wait for either the biopsy to be done or the results to be returned, especially if the patient has visual symptoms. There is evidence that several weeks of glucocorticoid treatment does not affect the biopsy results, so immediate treatment is the rule when the diagnosis is made.[5]

An elevated ESR is one of the most sensitive markers for temporal arteritis, and jaw claudication, diplopia, and an abnormal temporal artery are the most specific markers.

Using the ESR and the temporal artery biopsy result to assist in the diagnosis of temporal arteritis is a grade A recommendation. One study found that the combination of jaw claudication and diplopia was 100% specific for a biopsy with positive results. Treatment of temporal arteritis should not be delayed to await biopsy or its results. If there is a high clinical suspicion, treatment with steroids should be begun even if a biopsy has not been obtained. This treatment is a grade B recommendation.[7]

CLASSIFICATION CRITERIA

The American College of Rheumatology established a set of classification criteria in 1990 for temporal arteritis. A patient may be classified as having temporal arteritis by meeting 3 of the 5 following criteria: (1) age 50 years or older, (2) new-onset localized headache, (3) temporal artery tenderness or decreased temporal artery pulse, (4) ESR greater than 50 mm/h, (5) abnormal temporal artery biopsy findings of mononuclear infiltration or granulomatous inflammation.[15] However, these criteria were never meant for diagnosis. Patients without temporal arteritis can meet these criteria as can patients with other types of vasculitis. In one study, the positive predictive value of these criteria was noted to be only 29% when used on a population of patients in whom the disease is very low, such as in a primary care setting. The positive predictive value increases when the criteria were applied to a more select group, such as in a rheumatology practice. Therefore, these criteria must be used with caution when used as the sole basis for the diagnosis of temporal arteritis.[16]

DIFFERENTIAL DIAGNOSIS

The differential diagnosis of temporal arteritis involves several serious diseases. Multiple myeloma, leukemia, and other neoplasms should be ruled out in older persons presenting with fever, weight loss, elevated ESR, and vague constitutional symptoms.[12]

Because temporal arteritis can present as new-onset headache, the primary headache syndromes, including migraine headaches, cluster headaches, and tension-type headaches, should be included in the differential. The International Headache Society has criteria for the diagnosis of temporal arteritis as a cause of secondary headache. These criteria include (1) any new persisting headache, (2) at least one of the following: swollen tender scalp with increased ESR and/or CRP level or temporal artery biopsy showing temporal arteritis, (3) headache developing in temporal relation to other symptoms and signs of temporal arteritis, (4) headache resolving or greatly improving within 3 days of high-dose steroid treatment.[17] New-onset headache should also raise suspicion for intracranial mass or bleed.[7]

Pain in the jaw area could indicate a dental cause or temporomandibular joint syndrome. Pain in the face could indicate trigeminal neuralgia or sinusitis. Changes in or loss of vision could indicate a retinal vascular accident or cranial nerve neuropathy.[7,18]

TREATMENT

As soon as the diagnosis is established either by clinical and laboratory findings or by positive biopsy results, therapy should be initiated. Glucocorticoids are the first-line therapy for temporal arteritis at doses of 40 to 60 mg/d. The use of steroids has been a well-established therapy for many years and is a grade B recommendation. For those patients with visual symptoms, such as recent or impending vision loss, intravenous methylprednisolone, 250 mg every 6 hours, can be given for 3 days before changing to oral steroids.[7]

Symptoms of temporal arteritis respond rapidly to steroids, with many improving within a few days of initiation of treatment. The response to treatment is usually so dramatic that this rapid response is one feature of temporal arteritis in patients for whom histologic confirmation of the diagnosis is lacking.[19] Treatment with steroids may prevent vision loss but does not reverse it. If a patient does not respond to steroid treatment, reevaluation of the symptoms, examination, and diagnostic evaluation that lead to the diagnosis should be undertaken.[2]

Treatment is initiated in conjunction with an ophthalmologist to maintain close follow-up of vision changes. Also, temporal artery biopsy is performed if not done already to establish a definitive diagnosis of temporal arteritis. The initial dose of steroids is continued for 2 to 4 weeks or until symptoms have resolved and a normal ESR is achieved; then the dose can be tapered. Tapering is done with a gentle reduction of 10% of the total daily dose every 2 weeks until a dose of 10 mg/d is reached. The taper is then slowed to a reduction of the dose by 1 mg/d each month to avoid adrenal insufficiency.[5] During this time, ESR and clinical symptoms are followed to monitor for relapse or spontaneous exacerbation of the disease. An isolated increase of ESR alone is not a valid reason to increase the steroid dose, but this increase combined with worsening of clinical symptoms requires an adjustment of treatment. Rapid withdrawal of steroids can lead to relapse, but 30% to 50% of patients have spontaneous exacerbations, especially during the first 18 to 24 months of treatment. A treatment course of 1 to 2 years is often required, but some patients have a more chronic disease course and require low-dose steroids for up to 5 years.[2]

Aspirin should also be given to these patients to help avoid ischemic consequences of temporal arteritis. In 2004, a retrospective study found that patients who had been taking low-dose aspirin for cardiac reasons had lower rates of vision loss or stroke. Other studies have found similar results. Although no randomized controlled trials have been done, the use of low-dose aspirin (81 mg) to prevent temporal arteritis–related ischemia is a grade B recommendation.[7]

Treatment of temporal arteritis requires high dosages of steroids for months to years. High doses and long-term treatment with steroids inevitably lead to sequelae. Adrenal insufficiency can develop with abrupt cessation of steroid therapy, hence the extended taper. In cases of surgery, infection, or other periods of increased physiologic stress, stress doses of steroids may need to be given. Other common complications of the long-term use of steroids for the treatment of temporal arteritis include increased susceptibility to infection, hyperglycemia, glaucoma, psychiatric disorders, and impaired wound healing.[5]

Patients taking oral corticosteroids for a prolonged period are at increased risk for osteoporosis. The people with temporal arteritis typically are older (mean age of 72 years) and predominately women, making the incidence of osteoporosis more likely.[5] The American College of Rheumatology Ad Hoc Committee on Glucocorticoid-Induced Osteoporosis recommends that patients with newly initiated steroid therapy with the equivalent of greater than or equal to 5 mg of prednisone per day should take calcium (1200 mg/d) and vitamin D (800 IU/d) supplementation; make lifestyle modifications, such as smoking cessation and reduction of alcohol consumption; and initiate weight-bearing exercises. For those patients starting long-term glucocorticoid therapy of 3 months or more with the equivalent of 5 mg or greater of prednisone per day, bisphosphonates, such as etidronate and alendronate, should be added. These agents have been shown to be effective for both the prevention and treatment of glucocorticoid-induced bone loss. The committee recommends the assessment of bone mineral density for anyone beginning long-term steroid therapy and treatment with bisphosphonates for anyone with an abnormal T score. While on steroids, the committee suggests longitudinal measurements of bone mineral density as often as every 6 months to detect bone loss. In those receiving treatment for osteoporosis, yearly follow-up measurements are sufficient (**Table 2**).[20]

Several options have been proposed to try to avoid these complications of steroid therapy. One such option is the alternate-day administration of steroids. Several studies have shown that this regimen is less effective in achieving and maintaining remission. One trial also noted more patients with new-onset visual impairment when using alternate-day dosing of steroids. No changes to the current recommendations for treatment with daily corticosteroids have been made based on these studies.[19]

For those who cannot tolerate steroid side effects or have severe complications from steroids, methotrexate has been investigated as a steroid-sparing alternative. Several trials have been done with methotrexate to assess its usefulness in temporal arteritis to maintain steroid-induced remission, with conflicting results. A recent meta-analysis of 3 trials showed that methotrexate treatment decreased the likelihood of relapse when compared with placebo, but the magnitude of the effect was modest. It was estimated that the use of methotrexate saved each patient approximately 800 mg of prednisone over the total treatment course of temporal arteritis. However, no appreciable difference in steroid side effects was noted in patients, raising doubts if the amount of steroids able to be spared may not be truly significant. There seems to be a threshold of steroid sparing, which improves side effect and complication rates. More trials and longer study periods using methotrexate in temporal arteritis will need to be done before definite recommendations can be made regarding its usefulness in temporal arteritis as a steroid-sparing agent.[19]

A multicenter, randomized, double-blinded, placebo-controlled trial was done to assess the efficacy of blocking tumor necrosis factor with infliximab. This trial failed to show any benefit of infliximab over placebo in the maintenance of disease remission once it had been achieved with glucocorticoids and was ended early. A randomized placebo-controlled trial, including a mixed panel of patients with temporal arteritis

Table 2	
Prevention and treatment of glucocorticoid-induced osteoporosis	
New Therapy (prednisone≥5 mg/d)	Calcium (1200 mg/d) Vitamin D (800 IU/d) Lifestyle modifications
Long-term Therapy (treatment≥3 mo)	Calcium/vitamin D/lifestyle modifications DEXA scan at the start of steroid therapy and every 6 mo during steroid therapy Bisphosphonates (etidronates or alendronate or risedronate) If started on bisphosphonate medications, perform DEXA scan yearly
Steroid therapy and BMD T score below −1	Calcium/vitamin D/lifestyle modifications Bisphosphonates (etidronate or alendronate or risedronate) Monitor DEXA scan yearly

Abbreviations: BMD, bone mineral density; DEXA, dual-energy x-ray absorptiometry.

Data from American College of Rheumatology Ad Hoc Committee on glucocorticoid-induced osteoporosis. Recommendations for the prevention and treatment of glucocorticoid-induced osteoporosis. Arthritis Rheum 2001;44(7):1496–503.

and PMR, was completed using azathioprine. All the patients included had steroid complications. This trial demonstrated a modest prednisone-sparing effect, but mixing the 2 diseases makes interpretation of the results problematic. Statins have also been studied for their potential glucocorticoid-sparing effect based on their antiinflammatory effects and their benefits with regard to primary and secondary prevention of vascular occlusive events in atherosclerosis, with no benefits at low doses. More study is required on the use of statins at higher doses.[19]

DISEASE COURSE

Temporal arteritis normally runs a self-limited course of several months to as long as 5 years. Relapses occur most often during the first 18 to 24 months of treatment or within the first 12 months after the cessation of steroid therapy. Taper of steroids too quickly can lead to relapse during treatment, although spontaneous exacerbations can occur.[8]

A 5-year follow-up was done on 96% of the patients studied in the American College of Rheumatology Classification Study for Giant Cell Arteritis in 1990. Researchers found that mortality rates were virtually identical in the patients with temporal arteritis as in the general population.[7]

A potentially lethal long-term complication of temporal arteritis is delayed large vessel aneurysm. Thoracic aorta aneurysms were found to be 17 times more frequent in patients with temporal arteritis than in the general population and may not present until several years after diagnosis and resolution of other symptoms. These aneurysms are at risk for dissection and rupture. Lifelong yearly imaging of the thoracic aorta may be indicated to monitor for development of thoracic aortic aneurysm. CT and magnetic resonance imaging are the best imaging techniques to detect aneurysms or dissections.[2] Aneurysms were not found more often in those patients who had experienced more relapses or a more chronic course or had higher inflammatory markers at diagnosis. Therefore, the formation of the thoracic aortic aneurysms is believed to be a delayed consequence of the initial structural damage caused by the vasculitis rather than that of the persistent subclinical inflammatory activity.[19]

Temporal arteritis is a condition with serious morbidity if left untreated. The condition can present with vague symptoms, so physicians always need to be alert for the diagnosis when evaluating patients. The family physician should consider temporal arteritis for any patient older than 50 years presenting with new-onset headache or a new type of headache, abrupt loss of vision, prolonged fever, PMR, or elevated ESR. In the 1950s, before the introduction of glucocorticoids, as many as 60% of patients lost vision because of temporal arteritis. With the current standard of care therapy, only 15% to 20% of patients in a recent series have this complication. This statistic alone should point to the benefit that early diagnosis and treatment of temporal arteritis can provide.[19]

REFERENCES

1. Hellmann D. Temporal arteritis: a cough, toothache, and tongue infarction. JAMA 2002;287(22):2996–3000.
2. Salvarani C, Cantini S, Boiardi L, et al. Polymyalgia rheumatic and giant-cell arteritis. N Engl J Med 2002;347(4):261–72.
3. Vortmann M. Acute monocular visual loss. Emerg Med Clin North Am 2008;26(1):73–96, vi.
4. Unwin B, Williams C, Gilliland W. Polymyalgia rheumatic and giant cell arteritis. Am Fam Physician 2006;74(9):1547–54, 1557–8.

5. Meskimen S, Cook T, Blake R. Management of giant cell arteritis and polymyalgia rheumatica. Am Fam Physician 2000;61(7):2061–8, 2073.

6. Gabriel S, Espy M, Erdman D, et al. The role of parvovirus B19 in the pathogenesis of giant cell arteritis. Arthritis Rheum 1999;42(6):1255–8.

7. Donnelly J, Torregiani S. Polymyalgia rheumatic and giant cell arteritis. Clin Fam Pract 2005;7(2):225–47.

8. Epperly T, Moore K, Harrover J. Polymyalgia rheumatic and temporal arteritis. Am Fam Physician 2000;64(4):789–96, 801.

9. Salvarani C, Hunder G. Musculoskeletal manifestations in a population based cohort of patients with giant cell arteritis. Arthritis Rheum 1999;42(6):1259–66.

10. Norman D, Wong M, Yoshikawa T. Fever of unknown origin in older persons. Infect Dis Clin North Am 2007;21(4):937–45, viii.

11. Larson T, Hall S, Hepper N, et al. Respiratory tract symptoms as a clue to giant cell arteritis. Ann Intern Med 1984;101(5):594–7.

12. Schmidt W, Kraft H, Vorpahl K, et al. Color duplex ultrasonography in the diagnosis of temporal arteritis. N Engl J Med 1997;337(19):1336–42.

13. Schmidt W. Doppler sonography in rheumatology. Best Pract Res Clin Rheumatol 2004;18(6):827–46.

14. Karassa F, Matsagas M, Schmidt W, et al. Meta-analysis: test performance of ultrasonography for giant cell arteritis. Ann Intern Med 2005;142(5):359–69.

15. Hunder G, Bloch D, Michel B, et al. The American College of Rheumatology 1990 criteria for the classification of giant cell arteritis. Arthritis Rheum 1990;33:1122–8.

16. Rao J, Allen N, Pincus T. Limitations of the 1990 American College of Rheumatology classification criteria in the diagnosis of vasculitis. Ann Intern Med 1998; 129(5):345–52.

17. Headache Classification Subcommittee of the International Headache Society. International Classification of Headache Disorders, 2nd edition. Cephalgia 2004;24(Suppl 1):1–160.

18. Swannell A. Polymyalgia rheumatic and temporal arteritis diagnosis and management. BMJ 1997;314(7090):1329–32.

19. Cid M, Garcia-Martinez A, Logano E, et al. Five clinical conundrums in the management of giant cell arteritis. Rheum Dis Clin North Am 2007;33(4): 819–34, vii.

20. Recommendations for the prevention and treatment of glucocorticoid-induced osteoporosis. American College of Rheumatology Ad Hoc Committee on Glucocorticoid-Induced Osteoporosis. Arthritis Rheum 2001;44(7):1496–503.

Systemic Lupus Erythematosus: Safe and Effective Management in Primary Care

Joseph P. Michalski, MD[a],*, Charles Kodner, MD[b]

KEYWORDS

- Systemic lupus erythematosus • Diagnosis
- Primary care management • Primary care evaluation
- Hydroxychloroquine • Corticosteroids

OVERVIEW

The management of systemic lupus erythematosus (SLE) presents a special challenge to primary care physicians. The clinical manifestations of this "great imitator" are highly variable, and diagnosis requires clinical judgment, an appropriate degree of suspicion, and judicious laboratory testing. Patients with SLE can have acute disease flare-ups that require intensive treatment to prevent life-threatening complications, and their management often requires that multiple specialists be involved. The medications used often have narrow therapeutic indices, with many adverse effects.

However, many patients with SLE have relatively benign courses, at least in the early phases of their illness, and the management of their disease can be readily accomplished in a primary care setting. Some patients may have limited access to rheumatologists, and rely heavily on their primary care physicians to provide at least a presumptive diagnosis and initial management of their illness.

Although SLE is a complex illness, it can be diagnosed and managed to a large extent in a primary care setting with appropriate specialist care and involvement. Early diagnosis and treatment is beneficial for patients beyond short-term symptomatic improvement, in terms of reducing the risk of disease flares, although treatment efficacy must be balanced against drug toxicities. Inadequate treatment is frequent

[a] Department of Internal Medicine, University of South Alabama, 3301 Knollwood Drive, Mobile, AL 36693, USA
[b] Department of Family and Geriatric Medicine, University of Louisville School of Medicine, 501 East Broadway, Louisville, KY 40202, USA
* Corresponding author.
E-mail address: jmichals@usouthal.edu

Prim Care Clin Office Pract 37 (2010) 767–778
doi:10.1016/j.pop.2010.07.006
0095-4543/10/$ – see front matter © 2010 Elsevier Inc. All rights reserved.

before a diagnosis is made, during periods when a patient is lost to follow-up or is non-compliant, or in the early stages of a clinical flare when symptoms may be minimal. Also, because patients with lupus survive longer as a result of improved treatment options they are at an increased risk of chronic illnesses, including hypertension, hyperlipidemia, and cardiovascular disease, which require the monitoring and preventive care that is well known to primary care physicians. The goal of this article is to describe effective evidence-based diagnosis and management of SLE with a focus on the role of the primary care physician.

EPIDEMIOLOGY

Diagnosis of SLE requires maintaining an appropriate index of suspicion; in this regard, it is helpful to remember the general demographics and epidemiology of SLE. Lupus disproportionately affects minorities, especially African Americans but also Hispanics and Asians.[1] The great majority of patients are women, with a female/male ratio of 10:1. A recent study comparing long-term outcomes between adult- and childhood-onset lupus provides the age of onset data of a large cohort of patients living in the United States. The mean age of onset of 795 adult-onset patients was 36.5 years, whereas the age of onset of 90 childhood-onset patients was 14 years.[2] Most patients in both groups were of childbearing age. The overall population prevalence of SLE is 56.3 per 100,000 among adults older than 18 years.[3] In specific demographic groups, however, the prevalence among adults aged 15 to 64 was 100 per 100,000 white women, 400 per 100,000 black women, 10 per 100,000 white men, and 50 per 100,000 black men.[3] SLE can affect patients of any age, including children and the elderly. This article focuses on SLE in adults.

CLINICAL PRESENTATION

Early diagnosis and treatment of SLE can prevent disease flares as well as potentially irreversible damage to major organs such as the kidneys, lungs, heart, or nervous system.[4] Although there are many atypical presenting syndromes that may result in significant delays in diagnosis, most patients present with more easily recognizable disease patterns including joint pain and swelling, facial rash and/or photosensitivity, pleuritic or pericardial chest pain, Raynaud phenomenon and persistent fatigue, and fever or weight loss.

About 60% or more of the patients have skin and/or joint manifestations at presentation.[5,6] It is emphasized that the diagnostic criteria for arthritis in SLE include not just joint pain but some evidence of joint inflammation such as tenderness, pain on range of motion, or swelling, typically of the hands. The typical malar rash of SLE can be easily confused with other facial rashes such as rosacea and seborrheic dermatitis. Potentially helpful but not diagnostic features of the malar rash of SLE include absence of burning, itching, tingling, or other discomfort; the rash of lupus typically spares the nasolabial folds, a distinction specified in the American College of Rheumatology (ACR) criteria for SLE.[7,8] A substantial minority of patients present with pleurisy or pericarditis.[5,9]

SLE should be considered in the following situations, especially in women of child-bearing age:

1. Any subacute or chronic illness of unclear etiology
2. Significant proteinuria or cytopenias of unclear etiology
3. Recurrent or unusually severe venous thrombosis, or any arterial thrombosis
4. Facial rash or sensitivity to sun

5. Unexplained inflammatory arthritis
6. Pleurisy or pericarditis, congestive heart failure, or severe pneumonitis of unclear etiology.

ACR DIAGNOSTIC CRITERIA

The ACR has published a set of criteria for classification and diagnosis of SLE[7,8] summarized in **Box 1**. The criteria are clinical or laboratory manifestations of SLE, which distinguish, with reasonable sensitivity and specificity, patients with lupus

---

Box 1
ACR diagnostic criteria for SLE

The diagnosis of SLE requires the presence of 4 or more of the following 11 criteria, serially or simultaneously, during any period of observation.

Clinical Criteria

1. Malar rash: fixed erythema, flat or raised, over the malar eminences, tending to spare the nasolabial folds

2. Discoid rash: erythematous, raised patches with adherent keratotic scaling and follicular plugging; possibly atrophic scarring in older lesions

3. Photosensitivity: rash as a result of unusual reaction to sunlight, as determined by patient history or physician observation

4. Oral ulcers: oral or nasopharyngeal ulceration, usually painless, observed by physician

5. Arthritis: nonerosive arthritis involving 2 or more peripheral joints, characterized by swelling, tenderness, or effusion

6. Serositis: pleuritis, by convincing history of pleuritic pain, rub heard by physician, or evidence of pleural effusion; or pericarditis documented by electrocardiography, rub heard by physician, or evidence of pericardial effusion

7. Renal disorder: persistent proteinuria, less than 500 mg/24 h (0.5 g/d) or less than 3+ if quantitation is not performed; or cellular casts (may be red blood cell, hemoglobin, granular, tubular, or mixed cellular casts)

8. Neurologic disorder: seizures or psychosis occurring in the absence of offending drugs or known metabolic derangement (eg, uremia, ketoacidosis, electrolyte imbalance)

9. Hematologic disorder: hemolytic anemia with reticulocytosis; or leukopenia, less than 4000/mm^3 (4.0 × 10^9/L) on 2 or more occasions; or lymphopenia, less than 1500/mm^3 (1.5 × 10^9/L) on 2 or more occasions; or thrombocytopenia, less than 100 × 10^3/mm^3 (100 × 10^9/L) in the absence of offending drugs

Immunologic Criteria

10. Immunologic disorder: anti-dsDNA in abnormal titer; or presence of antibody to Sm nuclear antigen (anti-Sm); or positive finding of antiphospholipid antibody based on an abnormal serum level of IgG or IgM anticardiolipin antibodies, a positive test result for lupus anticoagulant using a standard method, or a false-positive serologic test result for syphilis that is known to be positive for at least 6 months and is confirmed by a negative result in Treponema pallidum immobilization or fluorescent treponemal antibody absorption test

11. ANA: an abnormal ANA titer by immunofluorescence or equivalent assay at any time and in the absence of drugs known to be associated with drug-induced lupus

From Tan EM, Cohen AS, Fries JF, et al. The 1982 revised criteria for the classification of systemic lupus erythematosus. Arthritis Rheum 1982;25(11):1274; with permission.

from normal individuals and patients with other disorders. These criteria were developed to identify patients for research studies, but they are commonly and appropriately used for clinical diagnosis as well. A patient is said to have SLE if 4 or more of the 11 criteria are present, "serially or simultaneously, during any interval of observation." It is noted that patients may have manifestations of SLE that develop later, and their diagnosis may not be evident until multiple criteria are present. For patients with less than 4 criteria, a diagnosis of "undifferentiated connective tissue disease" is preferable, because many of these patients never develop lupus.[10] At presentation, it is common for a patient to have only 2 of the 9 clinical criteria (in nearly any combination), with the diagnosis supported by a high-titer antinuclear antibody (ANA) and subsequently confirmed by the presence of one or more of the specific immunologic features such as anti-Smith, anti–double-stranded DNA (anti-dsDNA), or phospholipid antibodies. Primary care physicians can reliably use the ACR diagnostic criteria to make a presumptive diagnosis of SLE.

LABORATORY AND OTHER DIAGNOSTIC TESTING

Patients with clinical symptoms strongly suggesting SLE, such as arthritis or rash, may also have asymptomatic manifestations that can only be identified on judicious laboratory testing. In particular, early lupus nephritis or chronic hematologic disease (anemia, leukopenia, thrombocytopenia) is frequently asymptomatic. Although undirected laboratory evaluation is not recommended, if SLE is suspected, an initial evaluation including complete blood count (CBC) with differential, urinalysis (preferably including microscopic analysis), and measurement of serum creatinine level is reasonable. Other studies that should be considered are summarized in **Table 1**.

ANA AND OTHER ANTIBODY TESTING

The ANA test is highly sensitive for SLE but, depending on how it is done and interpreted, may have poor specificity. A positive ANA test result can occur in many other disease states as well as in a large number of healthy individuals.[11] In primary care practice, a great majority of positive ANA test results may be false positives, and represent either no illness at all or (less commonly) an inflammatory disorder other than SLE.

In this light, ANA testing should be performed in patients in whom SLE is suspected on other clinical and/or laboratory grounds such as those listed above. A negative fluorescent ANA (FANA) test result essentially rules out SLE.[7] The infrequent patient with

Table 1	
Further diagnostic testing for major organ involvement in early SLE	
Presenting Symptom or Finding	**Suggested Diagnostic Test**
Unexplained chest pain	Echocardiogram for possible pericarditis or pericardial effusion
Unexplained dyspnea or chronic cough	Chest radiograph, possible chest computed tomography, echocardiogram
Anemia	Reticulocyte count, RBC smear microscopy, Coombs test
Unexplained, significant proteinuria, hematuria, or RBC casts	Quantify urinary protein (urine albumin:creatinine ratio), consider biopsy to confirm lupus nephritis

Abbreviation: RBC, red blood cell.

a negative result for ANA by FANA usually has a positive result for SSA antibody.[12] If lupus is clinically suspected, ordering an SSA antibody as well as an FANA may speed the diagnosis. The most useful clinical information can be obtained by ordering an ANA by FANA with a titer rather than screening with an enzyme-linked immunosorbent assay test for ANA. Studies suggest that the latter test lacks sensitivity and specificity,[13] and that it provides neither a titer nor an ANA pattern to shed light on the patient's disorder and guide further testing. If an FANA is ordered, lupus is very unlikely if the ANA titer on a standard substrate has a titer of less than 1:160. The role of ANA testing is addressed further in another article in this issue.

If ANA is positive in a patient with compatible clinical features, the most useful additional tests are anti-dsDNA, anti-Smith, and serum complement levels. Anti-dsDNA and anti-Smith antibodies are very specific for lupus, and increased anti-dsDNA and decreased complement levels may indicate active lupus or an impending exacerbation of disease. Phospholipid antibodies, including lupus anticoagulant testing and anticardiolipin antibodies, should also be ordered. If elevated, they help confirm a diagnosis of lupus,[8] and indicate an increased risk of venous and arterial thromboembolic disease as well as possible pregnancy complications.

MANAGEMENT
General Aspects of Management

Having made a diagnosis, the initial challenge of therapy is to decide on an appropriate course of treatment with an immunosuppressive and anti-inflammatory regimen that adequately controls the disease manifestations while minimizing the risk of adverse side effects. This stage of management can be difficult because the manifestations of active lupus can vary from mild rash and arthritis to catastrophic life-threatening syndromes that require emergency treatment in the intensive care setting with the assistance of several subspecialists. However, the management of the most common presentations of SLE can be done in the primary care setting; including ongoing patient education, disease monitoring, and provision of other preventive measures to avoid complications of the disease or its treatment. This article emphasizes management of the most common presentations of SLE.

Physician-Patient Interaction

Effective SLE management requires a supportive and therapeutic physician-patient relationship with the primary care physician as well as the rheumatologist. SLE often affects otherwise young healthy patients for whom a chronic illness, with troublesome symptoms and potentially life-threatening complications, represents particular challenges. Denial of their illness or medications and nonadherence because of demands at work or in life may be particular issues with younger patients.[14,15] Some patients may be uninsured or underinsured[16] and may require additional support or resources to ensure medical follow-up, access to medications, and adequate monitoring of their disease.

Nonmajor Organ System Involvement

For milder lupus manifestations such as arthritis and rash, the mainstay of management is the antimalarial drug hydroxychloroquine (HCQ, Plaquenil). However, all patients with SLE benefit from antimalarial therapy, including those without symptomatic rash or arthritis. While HCQ is most clearly effective for treating skin and joint manifestations, it has broader benefits in terms of preventing disease flares and suppressing exacerbations of vital-organ involvement as well.[17,18] Although this drug has been in use for decades with well-known clinical benefits,[19] it may be unfamiliar to many primary care physicians and may be seen as a drug used primarily by specialists. However, HCQ can be safely and appropriately started in the primary care setting to ensure the most rapid and effective treatment, possibly while awaiting rheumatologic consultation.

The typical dose of HCQ is 400 mg/d (taken as 200 mg twice a day). The maximum recommended dose is 6.5 mg/kg to a maximum of 400 mg/d, regardless of the patient's weight. In general, HCQ is well tolerated by most patients, both acutely and long-term. During the first few days or weeks of HCQ treatment, some patients may experience symptoms related to mild autonomic nervous system effects, including dizziness, blurred vision, and gastrointestinal complaints of nausea, vomiting, or diarrhea. Should these side effects occur, patients should stop taking the drug until the symptoms completely resolve. If clinically necessary, HCQ treatment may be restarted at a very low dose, for example, half a tablet or 100 mg every 3 days, and then gradually increased to the appropriate dose over 6 weeks or more. Occasionally patients may experience rash or pruritus that necessitates permanent discontinuation of the medication.

The HCQ side effect of most concern is retinopathy, which is potentially irreversible. Retinopathy is relatively rare in patients treated with HCQ, contrary to the somewhat older drug chloroquine.[19] No cases have been reported in patients who have taken HCQ for less than 6 years, and only 47 cases have been reported between 1960 and 2005.[20] The risk of significant retinopathy is minimized by adjusting the dose of HCQ, depending on the patients' weight and monitoring for ocular toxicity with regular eye examinations. The frequency and method for screening eye examinations for HCQ retinopathy remains a subject of debate. Recent recommendations include a baseline examination and risk assessment within the first year of therapy, with no further screening indicated for the first 5 years for low-risk patients. Patients at high risk should be screened annually, and include patients with the following: daily HCQ dose exceeding 6.5 mg/kg; duration of therapy more than 5 years; age greater than 60 years; obesity; chronic renal, or hepatic disease; or concurrent retinal disease.[21] Maintenance therapy with HCQ is important not only for controlling the symptomatic manifestations of SLE but also for providing important long-term health benefits in terms of preventing complications of SLE and its treatment. All patients should be taking it if they can tolerate it.

Nonsteroidal Anti-Inflammatory Drugs

Nonsteroidal anti-inflammatory drugs (NSAIDs) are frequently recommended for 2 manifestations of lupus: arthritis/arthralgia and pericarditis.[22] Although NSAIDs may symptomatically treat SLE-associated arthralgia, they do not suppress overall disease activity. Thus, the well-recognized toxicity of NSAIDs suggests that exposure to these agents should be minimized. The adverse effects include gastrointestinal bleeding and peptic ulcer disease, cardiovascular toxicity, interference with the effects of aspirin in prevention of cardiovascular events,[23] and an increased the risk of myocardial infarction or strokes.[24] Many patients with lupus have apparent or subclinical glomerulonephritis and may be at increased risk of acute renal insufficiency or renal failure induced by NSAIDs.[25] For those patients with SLE whose joint or pericardial inflammation is associated with other manifestations that require corticosteroids, low to moderate doses of prednisone may preferable to NSAIDs pending the delayed onset of action of HCQ.

Corticosteroids

The risks of chronic corticosteroid therapy for lupus have been well documented,[26,27] but the benefits have not been quantified in recent controlled trials. Accordingly, recommendations about when to use corticosteroids and how much to use are somewhat a matter of personal opinion. Most patients with lupus require at least some chronic corticosteroid therapy, and oral prednisone is given most frequently. The goal of corticosteroid therapy for patients with lupus should be to use the lowest possible dose that suppresses manifestations of disease activity and prevents clinical flares. As a general rule, flares of active lupus are treated with higher doses of prednisone than the baseline treatment. When the active disease is controlled, the dose is tapered back to the baseline treatment required by that patient. The baseline dose of prednisone must be determined over time for each patient. Some patients with mild symptoms and no major organ involvement may be controlled on 5 mg or less of prednisone daily. However, many patients require 10 mg/d, and any attempt to reduce the dose much below that level results in a clinical flare. Consistent with this observation, a large multicenter analysis[28] found that one of the most highly predictive factors associated with new onset of organ damage was prednisone intake of less than 10 mg each day.

The dose of corticosteroids required to manage a flare depends on the type and severity of the manifestations as well as individual factors special to each patient. Mild flares of skin or joint disease may respond to a short course of low-dose prednisone (eg, 5–10 mg daily for a week or more) or an increase above their maintenance dose of 5 to 10 mg/d for a week or two or until the symptoms are controlled. Moderately severe nonmajor organ involvement (arthritis, dermatitis, serositis, and systemic symptoms) may respond to moderate doses of prednisone (eg, 20–30 mg daily). Corticosteroids should be tapered as tolerated, while monitoring clinical manifestations and laboratory parameters of activity until a maintenance level is achieved.

Preventing Complications from Corticosteroids

Patients with SLE on long-term maintenance doses of corticosteroids are at risk for chronic complications, primarily osteoporosis, accelerated coronary artery disease, and cataracts. Other complications such as poor glycemic control and femoral avascular necrosis may occur as well. Patients should be started on calcium and vitamin D at the time corticosteroid treatment is initiated. Typically, 1250 mg of calcium taken 2 or 3 times a day and 800 to 1000 units of vitamin D3 taken one time each day. A baseline bone mineral study should be ordered. The ACR recommends that all patients embarking on chronic treatment with more than 5 mg/d of prednisone should be started on a bisphosphonate regimen.[29]

Disease Monitoring

Especially early in the course of lupus, new manifestations may develop, so these patients should be seen frequently and have blood counts and urinalysis at those visits. At least for some patients, increasing titers of anti-dsDNA and decreased complement levels may precede a clinical flare. Early treatment with increased doses of corticosteroids may prevent the flare or reduce the total dose required to suppress the flare.[30,31]

Management of SLE Inadequately Controlled by a Combination of HCQ and Low-Dose Prednisone

This group consists of 3 categories of patients: those with systemic symptoms or mucocutaneous, arthritic, or serosal disease that cannot be adequately controlled;

those with vital organ involvement including moderate to severe nephritis or lung, cardiac, or central nervous system disease; and those with phospholipid-antibody–related disease. Vital organ involvement and the phospholipid antibody syndromes usually require subspecialty referral, and are discussed briefly later. Failure of the less serious manifestations to respond adequately to antimalarial and tolerable doses of prednisone (10 mg prednisone per day or less) should raise the possibility of starting one of the corticosteroid-sparing immunosuppressive drugs. The drugs most frequently used for unresponsive systemic complaints, or skin, joint, or serosal disease in SLE include azathioprine (Imuran), methotrexate, leflunomide (Arava), and mycophenolate mofetil (Cellcept). Some important details concerning these drugs are summarized in **Table 2**. Although many physicians may be reluctant to actually initiate treatment, primary care physicians, especially those in rural areas, should be able to monitor treatment started by a rheumatologist or other specialist.

Methotrexate and leflunomide are used mainly for arthritic symptoms and may reduce the dose of corticosteroids needed for systemic symptoms.[32,33] Azathioprine is the most broadly useful immunosuppressive drug for lupus[34] and may be the drug of first choice for nonarthritic manifestations of lupus unresponsive to antimalarial and low-dose prednisone. Azathioprine is also used to maintain cyclophosphamide- or mycophenolate-induced remission of vital organ diseases such as nephritis, cerebritis, and pneumonitis. All of these drugs except for azathioprine are teratogenic, and effective contraception is essential for their safe use. All of these medications increase the risk of infections, both conventional and opportunistic, and may increase the risk of malignancies as well.

Vital Organ Involvement in SLE

A detailed discussion of vital organ involvement in lupus is beyond the scope of this article, and most primary care physicians would seek subspecialty consultation for these problems arising in one of their patients. Nephritis is the most common vital organ affected in lupus. A substantial minority of patients have significant renal

Table 2
Immunosuppressive drugs frequently used as corticosteroid-sparing agents for patients with SLE

Drug	Usual Dosage	Common Side Effects	Monitoring Parameters
Methotrexate	7.5–20 mg every wk	Leucopenia, hepatotoxicity, pneumonitis, stomatitis, teratogenic	CBC with differential, LFTs every 4–8 wk, initial chest radiograph
Leflunomide	10–20 mg qd	Leucopenia, hepatotoxicity, rash, systemic symptoms, teratogenic	CBC with differential, LFTs every 4 wk
Azathioprine	25–150 mg qd	Leucopenia, hepatotoxicity	CBC with differential, LFTs every 4 wk
Mycophenolate mofetil	1.5–3 g qd	Leucopenia, anemia, hepatotoxicity, gastrointestinal symptoms, teratogenic	CBC with differential, LFTs every 6–8 wk

Abbreviations: LFT, liver function test; qd, every day.

disease at presentation and a majority have some evidence of renal involvement during the course of their disease.[35] Close monitoring of renal function, including urinalysis and creatinine, is recommended, especially during the early years of illness. Significant proteinuria requires further evaluation, and even a small elevation of creatinine suggests proliferative glomerulonephritis and an urgent need for nephrology evaluation and possible renal biopsy. Manifestations of lupus that affect vital organs or are life threatening usually require high or very high doses of corticosteroids. The dose and duration of treatment depend on the specific manifestation (eg, nephritis, cerebritis, or hemolytic anemia), the severity of the manifestation, and the patient's response to initial treatment. Immunosuppressive agents such as azathioprine, cyclophosphamide, or mycophenolate mofetil are usually given as well.

Pregnancy and Lupus

There are 3 major issues concerning patients with lupus and pregnancy. First is the risk of a clinical flare during the course of pregnancy or in the postpartum period. The second is the risk of complications, including fetal loss. The third is neonatal lupus. Although controversial, it is likely that pregnancy increases the risk of lupus exacerbations, especially in the third trimester and postpartum period. These flares can usually be controlled without excessive risk to the mother and fetus,[36] and pregnant patients can safely continue taking HCQ if they are on this at baseline.[37] Pregnancy is least likely to be associated with a flare if the mother has been in a remission for a substantial period before pregnancy. Flares and the risk of complications such as eclampsia are likely if the patient has active renal disease. The risk of fetal loss is greatly increased in patients with antiphospholipid antibodies. A combination of heparin and aspirin is given throughout pregnancy to reduce the risk of miscarriage and thrombotic events.[38] Anti-SSA and Anti-SSB antibodies cross the placental barrier to the fetus, and can cause neonatal lupus manifestations including heart block and rash.[39,40] In general, pregnant patients with lupus should be managed in a high-risk obstetric clinic and followed by appropriate specialists.

Antiphospholipid Antibodies

Antiphospholipid antibodies are associated with a greatly increased risk of thromboembolism and miscarriage in patients with or without lupus. About 40% of patients with SLE have these antibodies, and about 50% of those patients experience thromboembolism or fetal loss. Patients with lupus should be tested for the presence of these antibodies by ordering lupus anticoagulant and anticardiolipin antibodies tests. Treatment of the phospholipid antibody syndrome in pregnancy is described earlier in the article. The initial treatment of thromboembolic events for nonpregnant patients is heparin followed by warfarin. An international normalized ratio value of 2.0 to 3.0 is the goal. Prophylactic treatment with low-dose (81 mg) aspirin is probably worthwhile for patients with lupus with phospholipid antibodies who have not yet experienced a complication.[41,42]

Lupus-Related Emergencies

A detailed discussion of emergent lupus presentations is beyond the scope of this article, but a few suggestions may help the primary care physician recognize these situations early and initiate treatment while awaiting consultation or transfer of the patient. Some of the emergent syndromes include lupus cerebritis, transverse myelitis, diffuse pulmonary hemorrhage, hemolytic/uremic syndrome, and the catastrophic phospholipid antibody syndrome. These conditions should be considered if patients present with severe cerebral symptoms or paralysis, dyspnea and hemoptysis, hemolytic anemia and progressive renal failure, or widespread small vessel occlusions. Initial treatment with 500 to 1000 mg of intravenous methylprednisolone is reasonable in most situations. Many patients also benefit from intravenous IgG, cyclophosphamide, and plasma exchange or plasmapheresis.

SUMMARY

SLE is an autoimmune inflammatory disorder that most frequently affects women of childbearing age, especially African Americans. A diagnosis is made by confirming the presence of at least 4 of 11 criteria proposed by the ACR. A typical patient might have arthritis, a malar or discoid rash, and may test positive for ANA and anti-Smith or anti-dsDNA antibodies. The most common complication of vital organ involvement is nephritis. Virtually all patients should take HCQ and most will require corticosteroids. The dose of the latter should be kept as low as possible. Immunosuppressive drugs are frequently given as well, especially for vital organ disease. With better management, patients with lupus are living longer but are at increased risk of disease and treatment-related complications, including infection, cardiovascular disease, and osteoporosis. These problems should be monitored and treated in the primary care setting.

REFERENCES

1. McCarty DJ, Manzi S, Medsger TA, et al. Incidence of systemic lupus erythematosus. Race and gender differences. Arthritis Rheum 1995;38(9):1260–70.
2. Hersh AO, von Scheven E, Jinoos Yazdany J, et al. Systemic lupus erythematosus differences in long-term disease activity and treatment of adult patients with childhood- and adult-onset systemic lupus erythematosus. Arthritis Rheum 2009; 61(1):13–20.
3. Helmick CG, Felson DT, Lawrence RC, et al. Estimates of the prevalence of arthritis and other rheumatic diseases in the United States. Arthritis Rheum 2008;58(1):15–25.
4. Lam GK, Petri M. Assessment of systemic lupus erythematosus. Clin Exp Rheumatol 2005;23(5 Suppl 39):S120–32.
5. Heinlen LD, McClain MT, Merrill J, et al. Clinical criteria for systemic lupus erythematosus precede diagnosis, and associated autoantibodies are present before clinical symptoms. Arthritis Rheum 2007;56(7):2344–51.
6. Nossent J, Kiss E, Rozman B, et al. Disease activity and damage accrual during the early disease course in a multinational inception cohort of patients with systemic lupus erythematosus. Lupus 2010;19:949–56.
7. Tan EM, Cohen AS, Fries JF, et al. The 1982 revised criteria for the classification of systemic lupus erythematosus. Arthritis Rheum 1982;25(11):1271–7.
8. Hochberg MC. Updating the American College of Rheumatology revised criteria for the classification of systemic lupus erythematosus. Arthritis Rheum 1997;40: 1725.
9. Cervera R, Khamashta MA, Font J. Systemic lupus erythematosus: clinical and immunologic patterns of disease expression in a cohort of 1,000 patients. The European Working Party on Systemic Lupus Erythematosus. Medicine (Baltimore) 1993;72(2):113–24.
10. Mosca M, Baldini C, Bombardieri S. Undifferentiated connective tissue diseases in 2004. Clin Exp Rheumatol 2004;22(3 Suppl 33):S14–8.
11. Tan EM, Feltcamp TE, Smolen JS, et al. Range of antinuclear antibodies in "healthy" individuals. Arthritis Rheum 1997;40(9):1601–11.

12. Dahle C, Skogh T, Aberg AK. Methods of choice for diagnostic antinuclear antibody (ANA) screening: benefit of adding antigen-specific assays to immunofluorescence microscopy. J Autoimmun 2004;22(3):241–8.

13. Bernardini S, Infantino M, Bellincampi L, et al. Screening of antinuclear antibodies: comparison between enzyme immunoassay based on nuclear homogenates, purified or recombinant antigens and immunofluorescence assay. Clin Chem Lab Med 2004;42:1155–60.

14. Uribe AG, Alarcon GS, Sanchez ML. Systemic lupus erythematosus in three ethnic groups. XVIII. Factors predictive of poor compliance with study visits. Arthritis Rheum 2004;51(2):258–63.

15. Kumar K, Chambers S, Gorden C. Challenges of ethnicity in SLE. Best Pract Res Clin Rheumatol 2009;23(4):549–61.

16. Demas KL, Costenbader KH. Disparities in lupus care and outcomes. Curr Opin Rheumatol 2009;21(2):102–9.

17. Fessler BJ, Alarcon GS, McGuin G Jr, et al. Systemic lupus erythematosus in three ethnic groups: XVI. Association of hydroxychloroquine use with reduced risk of damage accrual. Arthritis Rheum 2005;52(5):1473–80.

18. Alarcon GS, McGuin G, Bertolli AM, et al. Effect of hydroxychloroquine on survival of patients with systemic lupus erythematosus: data from LUMINA, a multiethnic U S cohort (LUMINAL). Ann Rheum Dis 2007;66(9):1168–72.

19. Ruiz-Irasforsa G, Ramos-Casals M, Brito-Zeron P, et al. Clinical efficacy and side effects of antimalarials in systemic lupus erythematosus. Ann Rheum Dis 2010; 69(1):20–8.

20. Semmer AE, Lee MS, Harrison AR, et al. Hydroxychloroquine retinopathy screening. Br J Ophthalmol 2008;92(12):1653–5.

21. Marmor MF, Carr RE, Easterbrook M, et al. Recommendations on screening for chloroquine and hydroxychloroquine retinopathy: a report by the American Academy of Ophthalmology. Ophthalmology 2002;109(7):1377–82.

22. Horizon AA, Wallace DJ. Risk:benefit ratio of nonsteroidal anti-inflammatory drugs in systemic lupus erythematosus. Expert Opin Drug Saf 2004;3(4):273–8.

23. Farkouh ME, Greenberg BP. An evidence-based review of the cardiovascular risks of nonsteroidal anti-inflammatory drugs. Am J Cardiol 2009;103(9): 1227–37.

24. Graham DJ, Campen D, Hui R, et al. Risk of acute myocardial infarction and sudden cardiac death in patients treated with cyclo-oxygenase 2 selective and non-selective non-steroidal anti-inflammatory drugs: nested case-control study. Lancet 2005;365(9458):475–81.

25. Farkouh ME, Greenberg BP, Braden GL, et al. Acute renal failure and hyperkalaemia associated with cyclooxygenase-2 inhibitors. Nephrol Dial Transplant 2004; 19(5):1149–53.

26. Petri M. Monitoring systemic lupus erythematosus in standard clinical care. Best Pract Res Clin Rheumatol 2007;21(4):687–97.

27. Gladman DD, Hussain F, Ibañez D, et al. The nature and outcome of infection in systemic lupus erythematosus. Lupus 2002;11(4):234–9.

28. Toloza SM, Roseman JM, Alarcón GS, et al. Systemic lupus erythematosus in a multiethnic US cohort (LUMINA): XXII. Predictors of time to the occurrence of initial damage. Arthritis Rheum 2004;50(10):3177–86.

29. Recommendations for the prevention and treatment of glucocorticoid-induced osteoporosis: 2001 update. American College of Rheumatology Ad Hoc Committee on Glucocorticoid-Induced Osteoporosis. Arthritis Rheum 2001; 44(7):1496–503.

30. Tseng CE, Buyon JP, Kim M, et al. The effect of moderate-dose corticosteroids in preventing severe flares in patients with serologically active, but clinically stable, systemic lupus erythematosus: findings of a prospective, randomized, double-blind, placebo-controlled trial. Arthritis Rheum 2006;54(11):3623–32.

31. Bootsma H, Spronk P, Derksen R. Prevention of relapses in systemic lupus erythematosus. Lancet 1995;345(8965):1595–9.

32. Fortin PR, Abrahamowicz M, Ferland D, et al. Steroid-sparing effects of methotrexate in systemic lupus erythematosus: a double-blind, randomized, placebo-controlled trial. Arthritis Rheum 2008;59(12):1796–804.

33. Remer CF, Weisman MH, Wallace DJ. Benefits of leflunomide in systemic lupus erythematosus: a pilot observational study. Lupus 2001;10(7):480–3.

34. Abu-Shakra M, Shoenfeld Y. Azathioprine therapy for patients with systemic lupus erythematosus. Lupus 2001;10:152–3.

35. Ortega LM, Schultz DR, Lenz O, et al. Review: lupus nephritis: pathologic features, epidemiology and a guide to therapeutic decisions. Lupus 2010; 19(5):557–74.

36. Lima F, Buchanan NM, Khamashta MA, et al. Obstetric outcome in systemic lupus erythematosus. Semin Arthritis Rheum 1995;3:184–92.

37. Clowse ME, Magder L, Witter F, et al. Hydroxychloroquine in lupus pregnancy. Arthritis Rheum 2006;54(11):3640–7.

38. Ruiz-Irastorza G, Khamashta MA. Managing lupus patients during pregnancy. Best Pract Res Clin Rheumatol 2009;3(4):575–82.

39. Buyon JP, Rupel A, Clancy RM. Neonatal lupus syndromes. Lupus 2004;13(9): 705–12.

40. Lee LA. The clinical spectrum of neonatal lupus. Arch Dermatol Res 2009;301(1): 107–10.

41. Luzzana C, Gerosa M, Riboldi P, et al. Up-date on the antiphospholipid syndrome. J Nephrol 2002;15(4):342–8.

42. Lim W, Crowther MA, Eikelboom JW. Management of antiphospholipid antibody syndrome: a systematic review. JAMA 2006;295(9):1050–7.

Emerging Trends in Diagnosis and Treatment of Rheumatoid Arthritis

James T. Birch Jr, MD, MSPH*, Shelley Bhattacharya, DO, MPH

KEYWORDS

- Rheumatoid arthritis • Juvenile rheumatoid arthritis
- Disease-modifying antirheumatic drugs • Synovitis
- Elderly onset rheumatoid arthritis

EPIDEMIOLOGY

Rheumatoid arthritis (RA) is a chronic inflammatory disease with multiple comorbidities and is a cause of disability for many children and adults worldwide. The role of primary care is essential in early diagnosis and treatment of this debilitating disease. The prevalence of RA is estimated to be 0.8% globally, with women 2 to 4 times as likely as men to develop the disease. The incidence of RA in the United States is estimated at 25 per 100,000 men and 54 per 100,000 women, affecting approximately 2.1 million people.[1,2] Age at onset is usually between 30 and 50 years of age; however, juvenile RA and elderly onset RA (over age 65) also occur.[1,2]

In the United States, arthritis and other rheumatic conditions are the leading cause of disability. Approximately 39% of adults with arthritis report limitations in their physical activities because of their condition. Patients with RA are more than 7 times as likely to have greater than moderate disability as their sex- or age-matched counterparts. In addition, RA disability is linked with increased mortality. The Health Assessment Questionnaire (HAQ) disability index used to follow RA patients found that a change of 1 standard deviation in the HAQ correlates to an odds ratio for mortality of 2.3.[2] After 10 to 20 years of having the disease, as many as 80% show a compromise of their activities of daily living. Beginning early treatment can reduce the potential for disability by more than 60%.[3]

In economic terms, RA accounts for an estimated 250,000 hospitalizations and 9 million physician office visits annually. Within 2 to 3 years of diagnosis, 20% to 30%

The investigators have nothing to disclose.
University of Kansas School of Medicine, Department of Family Medicine, Division of Geriatric Medicine & Palliative Care, 3901 Rainbow Boulevard, MS-1005, Kansas City, KS 66160-0001, USA
* Corresponding author.
E-mail address: jbirch@kumc.edu

of those with RA become permanently disabled from work because of pain, impaired physical function, and transportation difficulties.[1,2] The total costs of arthritis and other rheumatologic conditions in the United States in 2003 was $128 billion ($80.8 billion from direct medical costs and $47 billion from indirect costs such as lost earnings). In addition, a reduced life expectancy of 5 to 15 years can occur.[3]

RISK FACTORS

Several environmental and genetic factors that potentially contribute to increased risk of developing RA have been identified. There are no definitive risk factors.

Environmental factors include hormonal exposure, tobacco use, microbial exposure, smoking, and consumption of more than 3 cups of decaffeinated coffee daily.[1,4] Among these, tobacco use has the most consistent evidence for an association.[4]

Genetic factors include female gender, positive family history, older age, and the HLA genotype.[1,4] In monozygotic twins, the concordance rate for the development of RA is more than 30%.[1] Siblings of patients with the disease are 2 to 4 times more likely to develop the disease than persons who are not related.[3] Among whites who have RA, 80% express the HLA-DR1 or HLA-DR4 subtypes.[1]

Risk of RA is reduced through high vitamin D intake, tea consumption, use of oral contraceptives, and with breast-feeding.[1] Women who have never given birth seem to have a slight to moderate risk of developing RA, and the evidence is mixed regarding an association between RA and hormone replacement therapy.[1]

PATHOPHYSIOLOGY

The pathophysiology of RA essentially remains only partially understood. A complicated interaction between environmental and genetic factors eventually results in the onset of disease. A viral infection or other biologic factor can initiate an abnormal autoimmune inflammatory response in persons who are genetically predisposed to RA. Where chronic inflammation exists in these cases of RA, there is an imbalance among the mediators controlling the system's response, resulting in eventual damage to cartilage and bone.[5] The pathophysiology of RA originates with inflammation of the synovium at any joint location, possibly triggered by the presentation of an antigen, autoantigen, or athrogenic peptide to the immune system. It appears that the subsequent cascade of inflammatory responses leads to proliferation of synovial macrophages, fibroblasts, and chondrocytes in the articular cartilage. These cells secrete enzymes that degrade proteoglycans and collagen, which eventually precipitate synovial tissue destruction.[5] Further infiltration by lymphocytes and other inflammatory cells occurs and is accompanied by angiogenesis in the synovium, causing irregular regrowth of the synovial tissue and eventually forming invasive pannus tissue. This process stimulates the increased activity of osteoclasts, resulting in further inflammation, leading to more cartilage destruction and the characteristic bony erosion of RA (**Fig. 1**).[1] Continued ongoing release of inflammatory mediators along with interleukins, tumor necrosis factor α (TNFα), cytokines, and proteinases, also contributes to the development of systemic symptoms and the extra-articular manifestations of RA.[1,5] There is suspected to be a "shared epitope," possibly derived from the disease-associated HLA-DR4/1 allele that is initially presented by an antigen-presenting cell to the T cell as a self-antigen.[6] Later in life, these T cells could be activated by cross-reactive antigens that display the shared epitope, leading to the inflammatory cascade.[6] Multiple infectious agents are known to possess potentially cross-reactive peptides so that possible reactivation of RA by these common and ubiquitous organisms might occur.[6]

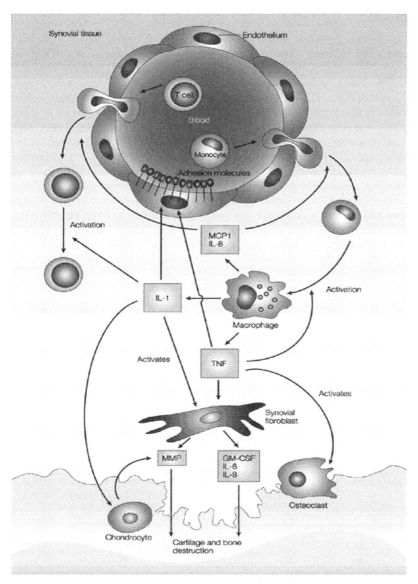

Nature Reviews | Immunology

Fig. 1. Pathogenesis of RA. (*Reprinted from* Pope RM. Apoptosis as a therapeutic tool in rheumatoid arthritis. Nat Rev Immunol 2002;2(7):527–35; with permission from Nature Publishing Group.)

Research continues to elucidate the role of macrophages and their cytokines in the synovitis of RA and to decipher the mechanisms of the apparent autonomous and aggressive behavior of fibroblast-like synoviocytes.[6] Greater understanding of these elusive issues could have a significant impact on the therapeutic approach to RA.

DIAGNOSIS

No single test confirms the diagnosis of RA. Diagnosis is largely based on clinical findings and patient history, which is challenging because the symptoms are similar to many other potential causes of joint inflammation and pain.[3] There are several tests that can be used to increase diagnostic probability and monitor disease progression. It is imperative that a diagnosis be established as early as possible, because a delay as much as 4 to 6 months in initiation of treatment could result in long-term joint injury.[5]

In 1987, the American College of Rheumatology (ACR), in conjunction with the American Rheumatism Association, established 7 diagnostic criteria to aid in the clinical diagnosis of RA.[5] These criteria are also used to define RA in epidemiologic studies.[4] Any patient who presents with at least 4 of the listed criteria for 6 weeks or longer is considered to have RA (**Table 1**).[7] Early RA is the classification of disease that is diagnosed within 6 months of symptom onset. There is considerable focus in this area because early treatment has been demonstrated to have a positive impact on disease progression and prognosis.[4]

Efficient diagnosis of RA requires vigilant attention to the patient's medical history.[3] Signs of early synovitis in the absence of obvious joint deformity might be uncovered by the squeeze test of the metacarpophalangeal (MCP) joints or the metatarsophalangeal (MTP) joints.[3] A key sign of RA at the time of the onset is symmetric joint swelling

Table 1	
1987 Criteria for the classification of acute arthritis of RA	
Criterion	**Definition**
Morning stiffness	Morning stiffness in and around the joints, lasting at least 1 h before maximal improvement
Arthritis of 3 or more joint areas	At least 3 joint areas simultaneously have had soft tissue swelling or fluid (not bony overgrowth alone) observed by a physician. The 14 possible areas are right or left PIP, MCP, wrist, elbow, knee, ankle, and MTP joints
Arthritis of hand joints	At least 1 area swollen (as defined above) in a wrist, MCP, or PIP joint
Symmetric arthritis	Simultaneous involvement of the same joint areas (as defined in 2) on both sides of the body (bilateral involvement of PIPs, MCPs, or MTPs is acceptable without absolute symmetry)
Rheumatoid nodules	Subcutaneous nodules, over bony prominences, or extensor surfaces, or in juxta-articular regions, observed by a physician
Serum RF	Demonstration of abnormal amounts of serum RF by any method for which the result has been positive in <5% of normal control subjects
Radiographic changes	Radiographic changes typical of RA on posteroanterior hand and wrist radiographs, which must include erosions or unequivocal bony decalcification localized in or most marked adjacent to the involved joints (osteoarthritis changes alone do not qualify)

For classification purposes, a patient shall be said to have RA if he or she has satisfied at least 4 or these 7 criteria. Criteria 1 through 4 must have been present for at least 6 weeks. Patients with 2 clinical diagnoses are not excluded. Designation as classic, definite, or probable RA is not to be made.

Abbreviations: MCP, metacarpophalangeal; MTP, metatarsophalangeal; PIP, proximal interphalangeal; RF, rheumatoid factor.

Adapted form Arnett FC, Edworthy SM, Bloch DA, et al. The American Rheumatism Association 1987 revised criteria for the classification of rheumatoid arthritis. Arthritis Rheum 1998;31(3):315–24; with permission.

with local heat and erythema. In the early phase there is usually no clinical evidence of joint disease and no evidence of cartilage or bone loss on plain radiographs. The physician or diagnostic clinician also needs to evaluate the patient for extra-articular features of RA, which will determine the potential course of the disease and guide treatment options.[3]

SYMPTOMS

Patients with RA typically present with pain and stiffness in multiple joints. However, one-third of patients have initial symptoms at a solitary location. The most common presentation of RA is that of an insidious onset of morning stiffness or diffuse aching that lasts for at least 1 hour or longer, followed by involvement of the small peripheral joints such as the MCP, MTP, and proximal interphalangeal (PIP).[3] It is not unusual for the larger joints to be affected first. Symptoms usually occur over weeks to months, yet in 15% of patients onset can occur more rapidly over days to weeks. Most patients have accompanying prodromal symptoms of weakness, fatigue, or anorexia. In 8% to 15% of patients, symptoms begin soon after a trigger event, such as a viral illness.[1] Characterizing the pain often helps distinguish RA from other forms of arthritis, as does a positive family history for RA. Determination of disability and ability to perform activities of daily living facilitates monitoring the effects of treatment.

The joints that are usually affected are those with the highest ratio of synovium to articular cartilage, such as the wrist, PIP, and MCP joints. The distal interphalangeal and sacroiliac joints are usually not affected. Affected joints are usually warm, tender to palpation, and boggy. There might be increased blood flow to the inflamed area with subsequent symptoms of puffy hands by patients.[1] Joint swelling is usually symmetric and, with tenderness on palpation, is one of the key signs of RA.[2] Beyond the joints, axillary, cervical, or epitrochlear lymphadenopathy may be noted. Muscles in close proximity to the inflamed joints often atrophy. Weakness is commonly out of proportion to the pain on examination. Joints are often held in flexion by patients to minimize painful distension of the joint capsules. Clinically, one may also appreciate decreased grip strength from tendon damage, tendon rupture in the wrist and fingers, decreased range of motion in the shoulders from synovitis and anterior effusions, and heel pain with antalgia from talus involvement. The hip is usually affected later, and hip involvement is usually rare.[3]

LABORATORY TESTS

Indications for testing include a history of persistent joint pain with early morning stiffness. Baseline laboratory tests are recommended and include a complete blood cell count with differential, rheumatoid factor (RF), and erythrocyte sedimentation rate (ESR) greater than 30 mm/h or C-reactive protein (CRP) greater than 0.7 pg/mL. Renal and hepatic function parameters are also recommended because findings guide medication choices, and monitoring should continue throughout the course of treatment.[1]

RF is an immune complex consisting of an autoantibody and IgG. A positive RF is not diagnostic of RA. Incidence of positivity increases with duration of disease (ie, 6–12 months), and with age. Of patients with RA, 20% may never have a positive RF, approximately 5% to 10% of healthy individuals are RF positive, and RF might also be positive in many other disease processes.[1,8]

Other laboratory tests that aid in the diagnosis of RA are as follows.

Anticyclic Citrullinated Peptide IgG Antibody

When positive, this test supports the diagnosis of RA. It is produced in the first stage of RA pathogenesis at the site of joint inflammation. During this process, citrullination of synovial antigens occurs, involving several synovial proteins. The antibody, anticyclic citrullinated peptide (anti-CCP), is secreted by B cells, which are present in the synovium and bone marrow of anti-CCP–positive patients.[9] Anti-CCP is more than 98% specific, and sensitivity increases when used in combination with RF. It might be negative during the course of early disease. One study found the anti-CCP antibody to be associated with some parameters of disease activity and severity, being more specific in patients with advanced RA with a mean duration of 9.8 years.[10]

Arthrocentesis (Joint Aspiration)

This option is a useful one if the diagnosis is uncertain. Arthrocentesis helps to differentiate crystal-induced arthropathies and septic arthritis. In RA, fluid is usually straw-colored, and fibrin flecks are often seen; clotting may occur at room temperature; a white blood cell count of 5 to 25,000 per mm^3 is common, with a differential count of 85% polymorphonuclear leukocytes. Findings also include no crystals, low glucose levels, and negative cultures.[1,8] Synovial fluid evaluation for anti-CCP has been suggested by a study to be a useful tool to assist with diagnosis of RA in cases of undifferentiated arthritis. The presence of anti-CCP in synovial fluid is a high risk factor for progression to RA.[9] Some patients may have negative serum levels when the joint fluid is positive.[9]

Plain Film Radiography

Plain film radiography remains the preferred method for initial examination to evaluate bone and soft tissue changes. Although a definite diagnosis might not be possible, even subtle findings and evaluation of soft tissue changes can facilitate a differential diagnosis. Depending on the severity of the disease, radiography can reveal soft tissue swelling and joint space narrowing as a consequence of cartilage thinning, or joint space widening as an indication of joint effusion. Juxta-articular osteoporosis is also one of the nonspecific changes that can confirm the clinical impression of an inflammatory process.[11]

EXTRA-ARTICULAR SIGNS AND SYMPTOMS

Although well described, the prevalence and incidence of many extra-articular features of RA are not accurately known.[11] It is also difficult to separate these findings into those that arise as a complication of the disease, its treatment, or an immunologic disease associated with RA but occurring in isolation.[11] Pathogenesis of extra-articular signs varies between patients and anatomic location of the findings, but it is reasonable to conclude that any component in the autoimmune pathogenesis of RA is associated. Extra-articular disease has a significant influence on mortality from RA.[11] Infection is the leading cause of death (25%), followed by cardiac and pulmonary disease (18%), with renal and gastrointestinal disease being equal but lower in frequency (10%).[11] Other manifestations of extra-articular disease are outlined in **Box 1.**

JUVENILE RA

Children are not exempt from the disease of RA. The true incidence is unknown.[12] A 2007 study by the Centers for Disease Control and Prevention estimates that

---

Box 1
Extra-articular manifestations of RA

Rheumatoid nodules of varying size and consistency are found in up to 25% of patients. Location: extensor area of the forearm (common), internal organs (rare). Complications: gangrene and ulcer formation.

Hematologic: normocytic, normochromic anemia; thrombocytosis or thrombocytopenia; lymphadenopathy.

   Felty syndrome: the association of RA with leukopenia and splenomegaly

Vasculitis: may involve eyes, brain, skin, renal, cardiovascular, and gastrointestinal (GI) tract

Pulmonary: pleural effusions, pulmonary nodules, interstitial lung disease, bronchiolitis obliterans with organizing pneumonia; complications of treatment with disease-modifying antirheumatic drugs (DMARDs)

Cardiac: pericardial effusions; valvular lesions; cardiac manifestations from systemic influences of RA such as serositis, amyloidosis, vasculitis, conduction abnormalities secondary to nodule formation

Renal: microalbuminuria (correlates with disease activity); mesangial glomerulonephritis; (nephritic syndrome); nephrotoxicity secondary to DMARDs

Ophthalmologic: keratoconjunctivitis sicca or secondary Sjögren syndrome; episcleritis and scleritis (prompt treatment necessary to avert vision loss); effect of drug therapy—risk of retinopathy with hydroxychloroquine requires ongoing surveillance

Neurologic: mononeuritis multiplex and central nervous system features including seizures, aseptic meningitis, and stroke secondary to vasculitis. Entrapment neuropathies via nerve impingement associated with subluxation of the atlantoaxial joint, amyloid deposits, or nodules

Musculoskeletal: osteoporosis and fractures caused by disease process and corticosteroid treatment. Muscular weakness of varying etiology

Amyloidosis: found in 21% of patients in postmortem studies of patients with RA

Data from Firestein GS, Panayi GS, Wollheim FA. Rheumatoid arthritis: frontiers in pathogenesis and treatment. New York: Oxford University Press; 2000.

294,000 children in the United States younger than of 18 years (1 in 250) have been diagnosed with arthritis or another rheumatologic condition.[13] The most common form of childhood arthritis is juvenile rheumatoid arthritis (JRA).[13] The American Rheumatism Association acknowledges 3 clinical classifications of JRA: systemic-onset disease (10%–20%), polyarticular disease (20%–40%), and pauciarticular disease (30%–40%).[12] Clinical symptoms are varied in each category and each type has its own unique presentation, clinical course, and immunogenetic association. The polyarticular and pauciarticular forms contain more than 1 subgroup (Polyarticular: RF-negative and RF-positive disease; Pauciarticular: early childhood onset and late childhood onset).[12] Recognition of the subgroups is important for the appropriate diagnosis and treatment of the younger JRA patient.[12] One feature that all JRA patients have in common is the presence of chronic synovitis.

Once treatment is initiated, children should be encouraged to lead full lives as much as possible. Occasionally, some may be disabled or too ill to be self-sufficient and require inpatient rehabilitation. Support and counseling is necessary to prevent educational deficits, provide support of career plans, and in general to prevent children from thinking of themselves as people with disability.[12]

Currently 75% to 80% of children with JRA are expected to survive the disease without disability.[12] Those at greatest risk for joint destruction are those with systemic-onset JRA and RF-positive polyarthritis. Careful follow-up is necessary for all JRA patients throughout the course of active disease, and there is always the possibility of unexpected recurrences even after years of remission.[12] However, the future remains positive for most affected children.

ELDERLY ONSET RA

Elderly onset rheumatoid arthritis (EORA) includes patients who develop RA between the age of 60 and 65 years. The prevalence is approximately 2% in this age group.[14] Symptoms of EORA are different from those in younger patients, and 3 subsets have been identified[14]:

1. Patients who have classic RA signs and symptoms with clinical onset similar to that in patients who develop seropositive RA at an earlier age. These patients have high levels of disease activity, and aggressive treatment is required.[14]
2. Patients presenting with symmetric arthritis associated with Sjögren syndrome. The synovitis is less severe and more readily controlled than in the first subset.[14]
3. Patients have a clinical picture that mimics polymyalgia rheumatica. RF is negative in the vast majority of cases but high levels of acute phase reactants are present. Arthritis in this subset of patients is usually well controlled with low-dose corticosteroid treatment; joint damage and radiological changes are less severe than in the other forms.[14]

EORA occurs in a balanced female to male ratio of about 1.5:1 to 2:1.[14] Poorer functional outcomes have been noted in patients who score high on the HAQ and who have RF seropositivity.[14] However, overall, EORA patients are more likely to experience clinical remission (odds ratio [OR] = 2.99) with a much higher remission rate in the seronegative EORA group than all other groups (including the younger seronegative RA group). It should also be noted that continuous use of corticosteroids for more than 3 months in EORA patients has been associated with joint erosion (OR = 4.09).

Diagnosis of EORA requires early and appropriate initiation of DMARD therapy no different from that given to younger RA patients. The higher remission rate in seronegative EORA patients implies that therapy might be given for a shorter duration than for seropositive patients. Awareness should be heightened regarding the increased risk of adverse events associated with RA treatments in the elderly patient. Careful follow-up and prudent use of the appropriate medications is extremely important.[14]

DIFFERENTIAL DIAGNOSIS

The differential diagnosis of RA is extensive. Most patients present with symptoms in common with RA. A careful clinical history, followed by a meticulous physical examination, and acquisition of prudent laboratory and imaging studies is mandatory to initiate the diagnostic process.[14] Differential diagnoses include but are not limited to the conditions listed in **Table 2**.[1,8,14] Potential causes of infectious arthritis include hepatitis B and C, human immunodeficiency virus, and other bacterial infections.

Included in the differential diagnosis for EORA is remitting seronegative symmetric synovitis with pitting edema syndrome (also known as RS3PE syndrome).[14] This condition historically develops abruptly in elderly patients with the finding of edematous symmetric arthritis involving the distal extremities, specifically hands and wrists and/or feet and ankles. The edema on the dorsal aspect of the involved areas is

Table 2	
Differential diagnosis of RA	
Connective tissue diseases	Crystalline arthropathy (polyarticular gout,
Fibromyalgia	pseudogout, chronic calcium
Other forms of arthritis (infectious, reactive,	pyrophosphate arthropathy)
viral, osteoarthritis)	Acute rheumatic fever
Seronegative spondyloarthropathies	Thyroid disease
Sarcoidosis	Still disease
Hemochromatosis	Polymyalgia rheumatica
Infectious carditis	Malignancy-related arthritis
	Hypertrophic osteoarthropathy

caused by extensor tenosynovitis. There is no development of bony erosions and RF is negative. Patients with the condition demonstrate a satisfactory response to corticosteroids, and the prognosis is excellent. It is still debatable as to whether this syndrome is part of the spectrum of RA or a completely different medical condition. Many of the same findings can occur in patients with polymyalgia rheumatica, other inflammatory arthropathies, and malignancies involving the hematologic system as well as solid tumors.[14]

TREATMENT

Early treatment reduces the rate of disease progression and is therefore recommended to be initiated during the early phase of the disease.[1] Many patients experience RA symptoms for an average of 9 to 12 months before a diagnosis is made.[2] The American College of Rheumatology Subcommittee on Rheumatoid Arthritis (ACRSRA) recommends that patients with suspected RA be referred to a rheumatologist within 3 months of presentation to confirm the diagnosis and initiate treatment. The National Guideline Clearinghouse also supports specialist referral and recommends urgent referral if the small joints of the hands or feet are affected, more than 1 joint is affected, or there has been a delay of 3 months or more between the onset of symptoms and seeking of medical advice.[15] Therapeutic goals must be discussed with the patient and should include preservation of quality of life, reducing pain, minimizing inflammation, protecting the joints, and reducing RA complications.[1]

Patients with mild disease and normal radiograph joint findings can begin treatment with hydroxychloroquine, sulfasalazine, minocycline, or methotrexate.[1,16] **Fig. 2** contains an algorithm that simplifies the approach to treatment.[1] Nonsteroidal anti-inflammatory drugs (NSAIDs) should not be used alone, as they do not change the disease course. Precautions should be observed with NSAID use, as RA patients are almost twice as likely as osteoarthritis patients to have serious complications from NSAID use.

Cyclooxygenase-2 (COX-2) selective NSAIDs are equally as effective as nonselective NSAIDs for reducing pain and inflammation as well as improving joint function. These agents should be used with caution in renal and geriatric patients.[1] There is also ongoing concern of the cardiovascular safety of COX-2 NSAIDs. Therefore, careful patient selection is imperative. There have been long-term studies, such as the CLASS study (Celecoxib Long-term Arthritis Safety Study), which showed a reduction in adverse upper GI events in patients taking celecoxib alone without low-dose aspirin versus NSAIDs alone or COX-1 versus COX-2 NSAIDs with low-dose aspirin.[17] Owing to the cardiac benefit of low-dose aspirin for patients with moderate or high

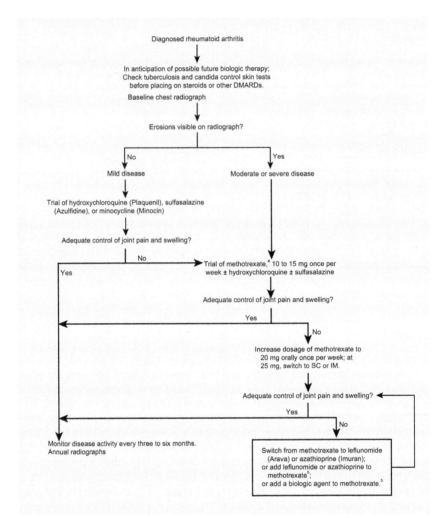

Fig. 2. Treatment algorithm for RA. [a]The following laboratory tests should be performed before methotrexate therapy begins, every 2 weeks for 6 weeks, then, if normal, every 2 months: complete blood count with differential, platelets, aspartate transaminase levels, albumin levels, and creatinine levels. When starting methotrexate add 1 mg oral folic acid per day to decrease side effects, and caution the patient to avoid alcohol. [b]When adding another DMARD to methotrexate, decrease the dosage of methotrexate to 10 to 15 mg once per week. (*Reprinted from* Rindfleisch JA, D Muller. Diagnosis and management of rheumatoid arthritis. Am Fam Physician 2005;72(6):1042; with permission.)

cardiovascular risk (Framingham scores >10%), a reasonable and proven strategy is to use a nonselective NSAID in combination with misoprostol or a proton pump inhibitor, instead of celecoxib, for patients on low-dose aspirin therapy who are at high risk for gastropathy.[18]

Glucocorticoids at dosages of less than 10 mg of prednisone daily are also highly effective to treat RA pain and stiffness, and can slow joint damage. Because of the multiple adverse effects of steroid use, dosages should be kept to the lowest needed to achieve therapeutic benefit. When discontinuing glucocorticoid therapy, a slow taper is recommended over approximately 1 month.[1] In addition, recent guidelines by the American Association of Clinical Endocrinology recommend supplements of 1500 mg of calcium and 800 IU of Vitamin D3 daily for patients receiving glucocorticoid therapy and bisphosphonate therapy for all adult women requiring more than 7.5 mg of prednisone or its equivalent for over 3 weeks.[19] When a single joint contributes to disability, intra-articular glucocorticoids are a safe, yet temporary option. Intra-articular injections can also be used as bridge therapy until DMARDs become effective, which has the potential to take several months.[5] Infectious causes should be ruled out before administering an injection.[1]

The recently published 2008 ACR guidelines for management of RA recommend using disease duration as a guide for treatment. There are 3 categories of disease duration: less than 6 months (considered to be equivalent to early disease), 6 to 24 months (considered to be equivalent to intermediate disease duration), and more than 24 months (considered to be long or longer disease duration). For biologic therapies, early disease is further subdivided by disease duration of less than 3 months or 3 to 6 months, when disease activity is high.[16] Most RA treatment plans include an NSAID for pain control with careful use of oral or intra-articular glucocorticoids and the initiation of a DMARD. Unlike past regimens, the ACR now recommends that DMARDs be initiated early in the disease to reduce progression.[16] Treatment protocols have been modified as a result of research demonstrating that joint damage begins early in RA, DMARDs have significant benefits when begun early, DMARD benefits are enhanced when used in combination, and new DMARDs are available with good therapeutic benefits.

The nonbiologic DMARDs addressed in the 2008 ACR recommendations are hydroxychloroquine, leflunomide, methotrexate, minocycline, and sulfasalazine. The biologic DMARDs included are abatacept, adalimumab, etanercept, infliximab, and rituximab. The remaining DMARDs are not included because they were not subjected to a systematic review of the literature due to their infrequent use (<5% of RA patients, eg, anakinra) and/or the high incidence of adverse events when they are used (cyclophosphamide, D-penicillamine, staphylococcal immunoabsorption column, tacrolimus). Abatacept and rituximab are the only 2 DMARDs that received an evidence-based recommendation (Level of Evidence for use: A). Disease activity (low, moderate, or high) and prognostic features are included with disease duration in evidence-based recommendations. Prognosis was defined as poor if patients had active disease with multiple tender, swollen joints, elevated RF, elevated anti-CCP antibodies, elevated ESR or CRP, and evidence of radiographic erosions.[16] Important predictors for a worse outcome include the presence of any of the aforementioned risk factors and poor physical functioning.[16]

DMARDs should be considered for all RA patients, regardless of stage. The DMARD agent of choice depends on age, compliance, disease severity, physician comfort, and comorbidities. Increasing evidence shows that DMARD combinations can be more effective than single regimens. Regarding the nonbiologic DMARDs, the ACR recommends the initiation of methotrexate or leflunomide therapy for patients with all disease durations and all degrees of disease activity. Hydroxychloroquine or minocycline monotherapy is recommended for patients without poor prognostic features, with low disease activity and with disease duration of less than 24 months. Sulfasalazine monotherapy is recommended for patients with all disease durations without poor prognostic features and with all degrees of disease activity.[16]

Those with radiographic joint findings and more severe disease should begin dual nonbiologic DMARD combination therapy. Methotrexate plus hydroxychloroquine is recommended for patients with moderate to high disease activity, regardless of duration or presence of poor prognostic features. Methotrexate plus sulfasalazine is recommended in patients with all durations if they have high disease activity and poor prognostic features. Hydroxychloroquine plus sulfasalazine is recommended only in patients with 6 to 24 months of disease duration and with high disease activity yet without poor prognostic features.[16]

Triple DMARD combination therapy of sulfasalazine plus hydroxychloroquine plus methotrexate is recommended for all patients with poor prognostic features and moderate to high levels of disease activity, regardless of duration of disease.

Regarding biologic DMARDs (anti-TNFα agents), the ACR recommendations are divided into those with RA for lass than 6 months and those with RA for longer than 6 months. The anti-TNFα agents are efficacious in improving disease activity, function, and quality of life when used alone or in combination with methotrexate or other nonbiologic DMARDs. Recommendations for the use of anti-TNFα agents with methotrexate are limited only to patients with early RA who have never received DMARDs, have had high disease activity for lass than 3 months, a poor prognosis, and without cost restrictions. In those with longer RA duration, the ACR recommends the use of anti-TNFα agents in patients for whom methotrexate monotherapy or combination therapy with nonbiologic DMARDs was inadequate.[16]

The risk of death from infection in patients with RA is approximately 6 to 9 times greater than in non-RA populations.[20] Risk factors for infections include corticosteroid therapy, comorbidities, skin breakdown, joint surgery, and established RA. Nonbiologic and biologic DMARDs and TNF antagonists may place patients at greater risk of infection. Therefore, when a fever presents in an RA patient, sepsis should be strongly considered and a rheumatologist should be consulted early during the initiation of care. However, patients on a DMARD and steroids may not mount a typical febrile response; therefore a thorough clinical examination is necessary, including a thorough joint examination in which joint pain might be the most significant sign of infection.[20]

The ACR recommends routine tuberculosis (TB) screening for all patients who are being considered for treatment with biologic DMARDs. This recommendation is based on the evidence of higher incidence of TB cases following the initiation of anti-TNFα therapy. All patients should be asked about their risk factors for TB. A negative TB skin test should not be considered an exclusion of latent TB infection because many RA patients are immunosuppressed. In cases of active or latent TB, anti-TNFα therapy can be started about 1 month after initiating anti-TB therapy with isoniazid.[16]

Contraindications to DMARD use include active bacterial infection requiring antibiotic therapy, active TB (untreated), active herpes zoster infection, RA-associated pneumonitis, or active life-threatening fungal infections. In addition, the ACR recommends against the use of biologic agents during a severe bacterial or viral upper respiratory infection. Each DMARD has its own monitoring requirements and contraindications that are discussed elsewhere.

Safety ratings vary for use of RA therapies during pregnancy. Methotrexate and leflunomide have been issued a safety rating "X" by the Food and Drug Administration. Safety ratings for other treatments include B for sulfasalazine, C or D for other nonbiologic DMARDs, and B or C for biologic DMARDS.

Several novel therapies have also been studied for RA. Statins (atorvastatin and pravastatin) may have anti-inflammatory properties in the synovium, with an ability to inhibit both the production and actions of CRP.[21] Other novel therapies that are being studied for the treatment of RA include hematopoietic stem cell transplantation and immunoadsorption.[21] Lastly, nonpharmacologic therapies must also be considered in RA treatment. These treatments include physical therapy, occupational therapy, patient education, and nutrition guidance.[22] Moreover, access to a multidisciplinary team is the best approach to improve symptoms, functional outcomes, and reduce the progress of disease in patients with RA.[15]

SUMMARY

RA is an autoimmune disease that is characterized by synovitis, which eventually causes destruction of cartilage and bone. The pathogenesis is still being elucidated by ongoing research, but is generally described by a complicated interaction of genetics and arthrogenic antigens in the environment that interact to precipitate an inflammatory cascade, leading to bone and joint destruction. The course of the disease is unpredictable and usually varies among those who are afflicted.[23] No single laboratory test or physical finding can diagnose RA because it is largely a clinical diagnosis. However, laboratory tests and radiologic findings when combined with the physical examination can help to increase diagnostic accuracy. Primary care physicians should include screening questions during routine visits to increase the early detection of RA. Patients who are diagnosed with RA by primary care physicians should be referred to a rheumatologist expeditiously to limit disease progression as well as to minimize the extra-articular disease involvement. If untreated, the great majority of these patients become disabled.[3] The recent development of DMARDs has had a positive impact on disease progression and patient outcomes. Conversely, their use can be complicated by the development of adverse reactions, which always have the potential to complicate the symptoms of disease. The onset of RA can occur at any point in the life span, so that attention to the history and physical examination is the best means of uncovering this potentially aggressive disease. Nonpharmacologic therapies are also an important component of treatment.

There remain several issues that primarily limit our ability to provide optimal treatment. Access to many therapies continues to be limited by formulary restrictions, the costs of the DMARDs, prior authorization requirements by private insurers (which often include the requirement for inadequate responses to multiple DMARD treatments), and further limitation of the more expensive DMARD therapies to individuals with the most severe and longest duration of disease.[23] Overcoming the barriers to optimal treatment requires the growth of awareness that the disabling and life-threatening elements of RA are comparable with those of many other diseases.[23] Despite the remarkable progress made in delineating the pathogenesis of RA, as well as the development of disease-modifying treatment modalities, many questions remain unanswered and the cure remains elusive.

REFERENCES

1. Rindfleisch JA, Muller D. Diagnosis and management of rheumatoid arthritis. Am Fam Physician 2005;72(6):1037–47.
2. Kountz D, Von Feldt JM. Management of rheumatoid arthritis: a primary care perspective. J Fam Pract 2007;56(10A):59a–71a.
3. Weinblatt ME, Kuritzky L. Rheumatoid arthritis. J Fam Pract 2007;56(4):S1–7.
4. CDC. Rheumatoid arthritis. Diseases and conditions 2009. October 28. Available at: http://www.cdc.gov/arthritis/basics/rheumatoid.htm; 2009. Accessed November 5, 2009.
5. Costenbader KH, Kountz DS. Treatment and management of early RA: a primary care primer. J Fam Pract 2007;56(7 Suppl):S1–7 [quiz: S8].

6. Arend WP. The pathophysiology and treatment of rheumatoid arthritis. Arthritis Rheum 1997;40(4):595–7.
7. Arnett FC, Edworthy SM, Bloch DA, et al. The American Rheumatism Association 1987 revised criteria for the classification of rheumatoid arthritis. Arthritis Rheum 1988;31(3):315–24.
8. ARUP. Rheumatoid arthritis. The physician's guide to laboratory test selection and interpretation 2009. Available at: http://www.arupconsult.com/Topics/RA.html. August 2009. Accessed November 5, 2009.
9. Heidari B, Abedi H, Firouzjahi A, et al. Diagnostic value of synovial fluid anti-cyclic citrullinated peptide antibody for rheumatoid arthritis. Rheumatol Int October 13, 2009. [online].
10. Samanci N, Ozdem S, Akbas H, et al. Diagnostic value and clinical significance of anti-CCP in patients with advanced rheumatoid arthritis. J Natl Med Assoc 2005;97(8):1120–6.
11. Firestein GS, Panayi GS, Wollheim FA. Rheumatoid arthritis: frontiers in pathogenesis and treatment. New York: Oxford University Press; 2000.
12. Schaller JG. Juvenile rheumatoid arthritis. Pediatr Rev 1997;18(10):337–49.
13. CDC. Centers for Disease Control and Prevention. Childhood arthritis. 2009. Available at: http://www.cdc.gov/arthritis/basics/childhood.htm. Accessed December 2, 2009.
14. Villa-Blanco JI, Calvo-Alen J. Elderly onset rheumatoid arthritis: differential diagnosis and choice of first-line and subsequent therapy. Drugs Aging 2009;26(9):739–50.
15. National Guideline Clearinghouse. Rheumatoid Arthritis. The management of rheumatoid arthritis in adults. 2003 November (revised 2009 February). NGC:007178. Available at: www.guideline.gov. Accessed October 15, 2009.
16. Saag KG, Teng GG, Patkar NM, et al. American College of Rheumatology 2008 recommendations for the use of nonbiologic and biologic disease-modifying antirheumatic drugs in rheumatoid arthritis. Arthritis Rheum 2008;59(6):762–84.
17. Silverstein F, Faich G, Goldstein JL, et al. Gastrointestinal toxicity with celecoxib vs nonsteroidal anti-inflammatory drugs for osteoarthritis and rheumatoid arthritis: the CLASS study: a randomized controlled trial. Celecoxib long-term arthritis safety study. JAMA 2000;284(10):1247–55.
18. Lo V, Meadows SE, Saseen J. When should COX-2 selective NSAIDs be used for osteoarthritis and rheumatoid arthritis? J Fam Pract 2006;55(3):260–2.
19. Hodgson SF, Watts NB, Bilezikian JP, et al, AACE Osteoporosis Task Force. American Association of Clinical Endocrinologists medical guidelines for the clinical practice for the prevention and treatment of postmenopausal osteoporosis. Endocr Pract 2003;9(6):544–64.
20. Bingham CO 3rd, Miner MM. Treatment, management, and monitoring of established rheumatoid arthritis. J Fam Pract 2007;56(Suppl Rapid 10):S1–7 [quiz: S8].
21. Harris E. Miscellaneous novel therapies in rheumatoid arthritis. Waltham (MA): UpToDate, Inc; 2009.
22. Harris E. Nonpharmacologic and preventive therapies of rheumatoid arthritis. Waltham (MA): UpToDate, Inc; 2009.
23. Bykerk V. Unmet needs in rheumatoid arthritis. J Rheumatol Suppl 2009;82:42–6.

Surveillance for and Prevention of Nonrheumatologic Diseases in the Patient with a Rheumatologic Diagnosis

Ehab A. Molokhia, MD[a,b,*]

KEYWORDS

• Rheumatology • Surveillance • Monitoring • Adverse events
• Investigations

Primary care physicians encounter numerous patients diagnosed with rheumatologic diseases, both systemic and localized, daily in their offices. Although many patients with systemic illness are followed up by rheumatologists, the primary care physician is frequently expected to assist with, if not assume, the care of these patients and is often the sole provider of care for patients with localized illness. Therefore, the primary care physician must monitor the complications of the disease process and their effects on different organ systems, and be aware of the patient's drug regimen and potential adverse reactions.

The medications used in the treatment of different rheumatologic diseases, while effective, are often associated with toxic effects on the human body. In 1992, an international collaborative group known as Outcome Measures in Rheumatoid Arthritis Clinical Trials (OMERACT) was formed in response to the need to form consistency in obtaining information regarding adverse events, severity ratings, time frames, and judgment regarding causation. The collaborative group currently tracks adverse events and attributes to aid in toxicity assessment and patient satisfaction.[1,2] The work of this group informs much of the guidelines surrounding the use of medications in rheumatologic illnesses.

[a] Department of Family Medicine, University of South Alabama, 1504 Springhill Avenue, Suite 3414, Mobile, AL 36604, USA
[b] USA Family Practice Clinic, Mobile, AL, USA
* Department of Family Medicine, University of South Alabama, 1504 Springhill Avenue, Suite 3414, Mobile, AL 36604.
E-mail address: emolokhia@usouthal.edu

Prim Care Clin Office Pract 37 (2010) 793–804
doi:10.1016/j.pop.2010.07.009
0095-4543/10/$ – see front matter © 2010 Elsevier Inc. All rights reserved.

SURVEILLANCE IN COMMON RHEUMATOLOGIC DISEASES
Cardiovascular Disease

Many systemic rheumatic illnesses are associated with increased age-adjusted mortality, mostly as a consequence of coronary artery disease. Prospective studies have shown that rheumatoid arthritis (RA) is associated with a doubling of the risk of coronary artery disease or myocardial infarction.[3] Women aged 35 to 44 years with systemic lupus erythematosus (SLE) have a 50 times greater chance of developing a myocardial infarction. Hyperlipidemia caused by nephrotic syndrome is thought to be one of the causes of this increased rate, but the inflammatory disease process is implicated as well. Increased homocysteine levels (>14·1 μmol/L in up to 15% of the patients with SLE) as well as the increased incidence of hypertension caused by the use of glucocorticoids in the treatment of SLE are also associated with higher incidence of cardiovascular disease.[4] It is suspected that other inflammatory arthropathies may also be associated with increased risk, although the mechanism is yet to be determined. In patients with inflammatory arthropathies, it is prudent to err on the side of tight lipid management and aggressive risk factor modification to prevent accelerated coronary artery disease. In addition, in diseases in which the administration of disease-modifying antirheumatic drugs (DMARDs) is indicated, initiation may retard the development of plaque.[5]

Renal Disease

Many rheumatologic illnesses also have renal disease as a consequence, as a result of illness progression as well as complications of treatment. In RA, for example, it has been reported that between 5% and 50% of patients have chronic renal disease.[6] Proteinuria is usually the first sign, developing 6 to 12 months after initiation of therapy; however, discontinuation of the offending therapy leads to the resolution of proteinuria in most cases after 9 to 12 months. Secondary amyloidosis is also another rare complication of RA, and its incidence has markedly decreased with the availability of effective medications for therapy. Lupus is also strongly associated with renal disease, as a consequence of both the illness and the treatment. In addition, many patients with rheumatologic complaints are on long-term nonsteroidal therapy, both prescribed and obtained over the counter. Because many of these patients are on potentially nephrotoxic regimens and have the potential of progression because of worsening of illness, it is reasonable that these individuals be considered at high risk and monitored periodically with spot urine test for microalbumin and serum creatinine measurements.

Osteoporosis

Management of rheumatologic illnesses often incorporates medications that are associated with bone loss. In addition, the illness may also lead to bone loss. The risk of bone loss is further increased with the presence of other known risk factors for the development of osteoporosis, such as age, family history, menopause, increased alcohol consumption, and decreased weight-bearing activities. Adherence to screening protocols with a dual-energy x-ray absorptiometry (DXA) scan is important to aid in the early detection and prevention of sequelae such as fractures. Calcium supplementation is also important (calcium, 1500 mg, and vitamin D_3, 800 IU, daily). Patients on long-term therapy with glucocorticoids (prednisone, more than 5 mg, or its equivalent for 3 weeks) should be on a bisphosphonate concurrently.[7]

Malignancies

Some patients with rheumatic diseases have a higher incidence of cancer. This phenomenon has not only been linked to some of the medications used to treat the disease process, as discussed earlier, but also to the underlying disease process. For example, patients with dermatomyositis or polymyositis have had a higher incidence of cancers of the breast, uterus, and ovaries in women as well as cancers of the lung, prostate, and digestive tract in men. Also, the incidence of hematologic malignancies is high in both sexes. The relative risk of developing cancer ranges between 2.4 and 4.4 and 1.7 and 2.1 in female and male patients, respectively when compared with the general population. Patients with RA have shown an increased risk of developing Hodgkin and non–Hodgkin lymphoma as well as a possible increased risk of developing multiple myeloma and leukemia. An association between systemic sclerosis and lung, breast, hematopoietic, and lymphoproliferative malignancies has been demonstrated, with an overall risk of cancer between 1.5 and 2.4.[8] There is an increased risk of developing non–Hodgkin lymphoma in patients with Sjögren syndrome, with the prevalence reaching up to 4% to 10% in patients followed up for 10 years or more. The risk of developing non–Hodgkin lymphoma has been estimated to be 44 times higher than in the general population.[8]

Although the risk of cancer in patients with certain rheumatic diseases has been higher than that of the general population, no clear recommendations have been put forth for cancer screening for these patients. With the exception of the guidelines for patients who were prescribed cyclophosphamide (CYC), it is important for the primary care physician to strictly adhere to cancer screening guidelines of the United States Preventive Services Task Force and the American Cancer Society. The primary care provider should also be vigilant for signs and symptoms of associated cancers when caring for patients with rheumatologic illness.

SURVEILLANCE AND DRUG THERAPY

The American College of Rheumatology has put forth some guidelines to assist practitioners in monitoring patients on antirheumatic drugs. These recommendations are mainly based on the concerns associated with several drugs and their documented adverse reactions and toxicities. However, other considerations in their guidelines include patient convenience, for example, the number of phlebotomies proposed, as well as cost-effectiveness and the number of office visits. Hence, the intervals of monitoring patients are based on expert consensus to a great extent. **Tables 1–3** suggest the periodicity of testing based on available evidence.

DMARDs

DMARDs are given to most patients who have a confirmed diagnosis of RA, which is especially the case for nonbiologic DMARDs. However, with the emergence of newer classes, biologic DMARDs are being prescribed at an increasing frequency. Fewer data are available regarding the possible adverse effects of the biologic DMARDs, which renders the establishment of well-defined monitoring guidelines difficult.

With the initiation of DMARDs, whether biologic or nonbiologic, it is commonly recommended to obtain baseline laboratory profiles to include a complete blood cell count (CBC), and levels of liver transaminases and serum creatinine (level of evidence B). These profiles were recommended by a task force panel (TFP) of internationally recognized clinicians chosen for their expertise in the use of DMARDs, methodologists, and patient representatives. In addition, the TFP recommended the screening for both hepatitis B and C in higher-risk populations when initiating

Table 1
Recommended baseline assessment before starting antirheumatic therapy, obtained from the American College of Rheumatology

Therapeutic Agent	Baseline Investigations Before Initiation of Therapy									
	CBC	Liver Transaminases	Albumin	Serum Creatinine	Hepatitis B and C Testing	Eye Examination	CXR	PPD	Urinalysis	Others
Hydroxychloroquine	◆	◆		◆		◆				
Leflunomide	◆	◆	◆	◆	◆					
Methotrexate	◆	◆	◆	◆	◆		◆			
Minocycline	◆	◆		◆						
Sulfasalazine	◆	◆	◆	◆					◆	Urine protein
Azathioprine	◆	◆	◆	◆						
Intramuscular Gold	◆			◆					◆	Urine protein
Oral Gold	◆								◆	Urine protein
Cyclosporin	◆	◆	◆	◆						Uric acid, Blood pressure
CYC	◆	◆		◆					◆	
Etanercept							◆	◆		
Kineret							◆	◆		
Infliximab							◆	◆		
Adalimumab							◆	◆		
Glucocorticoids										Chemistry, Blood pressure
NSAIDs	◆	◆		◆					◆	

Abbreviations: CXR, chest radiograph; NSAIDs, nonsteroidal anti-inflammatory drugs; PPD, purified protein derivative.

Data from Saag KG, Teng GG, Patkar NM, et al. American College of Rheumatology 2008 recommendations for the use of nonbiologic and biologic disease-modifying antirheumatic drugs in rheumatoid arthritis. Arthritis Rheum 2008;59(6):762–84; and Guidelines for referral and management of systemic lupus erythematosus in adults. American College of Rheumatology Ad Hoc Committee on Systemic Lupus Erythematosus Guidelines. Arthritis Rheum 1999;42(9):1785–96.

Table 2
Recommended baseline assessment for starting antirheumatic therapy, obtained from the American College of Rheumatology

Therapeutic Agent	Initial Laboratory Monitoring After Initiation of Therapy
Hydroxychloroquine	None
Leflunomide	CBC, levels of liver transaminases, CP8 every 2–4 wk for the first 3 mo
Methotrexate	CBC, levels of liver transaminases, CP8 every 2–4 wk for the first 3 mo
Minocycline	None
Sulfasalazine	CBC, levels of liver transaminases, CP8 every 2–4 wk for the first 3 mo
Azathioprine	CBC every 1–2 wk initially and with every change of dose
Intramuscular gold	CBC & urine dipstick every 1–2 wk for the first 20 wk
Oral gold	None
Cyclosporin	Levels of creatinine every 2 wk until the dose is stable
CYC	CBC every 1–2 wk with change of dose
Etanercept Kineret Infliximab Adalimumab Glucocorticoids	No evidence, recommend investigations and monitoring based on reasonable care and patient symptoms
NSAIDs	Levels of serum creatinine weekly for 3 wk for patients on ACE inhibitors or diuretics

Abbreviations: ACE, angiotensin-converting enzyme; CP8, chemistry panel 8; NSAIDs, nonsteroidal anti-inflammatory drugs.

Data from Saag KG, Teng GG, Patkar NM, et al. American College of Rheumatology 2008 recommendations for the use of nonbiologic and biologic disease-modifying antirheumatic drugs in rheumatoid arthritis. Arthritis Rheum 2008;59(6):762–84; and Guidelines for referral and management of systemic lupus erythematosus in adults. American College of Rheumatology Ad Hoc Committee on Systemic Lupus Erythematosus Guidelines. Arthritis Rheum 1999;42(9):1785–96.

leflunomide and methotrexate. Influenza vaccination is recommended for all patients in whom the use of both biologic and nonbiologic DMARDs is initiated. Pneumococcal vaccination is also recommended for patients starting leflunomide, methotrexate, or sulfasalazine and biologic DMARDs if they are not previously immunized, because of an associated increased risk of respiratory tract infections, and vaccination should be repeated every 5 years.[9,10] Other patients at a higher risk for developing hepatitis B should be offered the vaccine as well. Live vaccines, such as those used for measles, rubella, and mumps, are contraindicated in patients on biologic DMARDs. Patients starting therapy with hydroxychloroquine should receive an ophthalmologic examination within the first year of therapy to include a retinal examination and testing of central visual field sensitivity. If the patient's test results are found to be normal and the patient is in a low-risk category (no retinal or liver disease and younger than 60 years), repeat testing may be extended to 5 years as per recommendations of the American Academy of Ophthalmology. High-risk patients will continue to require eye examinations every 6 to 12 months.

After initiation, or after a significant increase in dosage of leflunomide, methotrexate, or sulfasalazine, the TFP recommends obtaining CBC and assessing levels of liver transaminases and serum creatinine every 2 to 4 weeks for the following 3 months, every 8 to 12 weeks for the next 3 months, and every 12 weeks after 6 months of therapy, if the therapy is deemed stable. No surveillance testing was recommended for patients taking hydroxychloroquine or minocycline.

Table 3
Recommended ongoing laboratory monitoring (in months) for antirheumatic therapy, obtained from the American College of Rheumatology

Ongoing Monitoring	CBC	Liver Transaminases	Albumin	Serum Creatinine	Urinalysis	Others
Hydroxychloroquine						Fundoscopic examination annually
Leflunomide	3	3	3	3		
Methotrexate	3	3	3	3		
Minocycline						
Sulfasalazine	3	3		3		
Azathioprine	3					
Intramuscular gold	2				2	
Oral gold	3				3	
Cyclosporin				1		
CYC	1				1	Urinalysis annually after cessation
Etanercept						
Kineret		No evidence, recommend investigations and monitoring based on reasonable care and patient symptoms				
Infliximab						
Adalimumab						
Glucocorticoids						Examination of urine or estimating blood glucose levels annually
NSAIDs	12			12		

Abbreviation: NSAIDs, nonsteroidal anti-inflammatory drugs.
Data from Saag KG, Teng GG, Patkar NM, et al. American College of Rheumatology 2008 recommendations for the use of nonbiologic and biologic disease-modifying antirheumatic drugs in rheumatoid arthritis. Arthritis Rheum 2008;59(6):762–84; and Guidelines for referral and management of systemic lupus erythematosus in adults. American College of Rheumatology Ad Hoc Committee on Systemic Lupus Erythematosus Guidelines. Arthritis Rheum 1999;42(9):1785–96.

Biologic DMARDs and Tuberculosis Screening

An increased incidence of tuberculosis (TB) has been documented in patients taking anti–tumor necrosis factor α (anti–TNF-α), a subcategory of biologic DMARDs. Consequently, the TFP has recommended routine TB screening for patients before initiating biologic DMARD therapy. It should be noted that patients with RA have immunosuppression, which may increase the likelihood of false-negative results. It is therefore important to take a careful history for previous exposures or other risk factors; in such cases, further imaging studies may be warranted. In actual practice, surveillance may not be done as often as it should be. In 2002, a survey of rheumatologists revealed that 83% ordered a purified protein derivative (PPD) test before initiation of therapy but only 50% ordered a chest radiograph, which is recommended if the PPD test result is positive.[11]

Anti–TNF-α

In one study, anti–TNF-α therapy has been associated with a doubling of the risk of other serious infections.[12] Another observational study from a German registry that included 512 patients treated with etanercept and 346 patients treated with infliximab also revealed an increased risk. The adjusted relative risk of a moderate or severe infection was 3.0 (95% confidence interval [CI] 1.8–5.1) for infliximab and 2.3 (95% CI 1.4–3.9) for etanercept when compared with conventional DMARDs.[13]

Hydroxychloroquine

Hydroxychloroquine, an antimalarial drug used in the treatment of RA, has a relatively safe side effect profile, with serious adverse events occurring rarely. The most common side effects involve the gastrointestinal system, with nausea being the predominant symptom. Vomiting and diarrhea may also occur. Other effects caused by the drug include headaches, neuropathy, skeletal myopathy, and cardiomyopathy.

As discussed earlier, ocular effects are of particular significance in monitoring patients taking hydroxychloroquine. Corneal deposits are rare but may occur, especially when taking doses higher than 400 mg/d. However, these deposits do not affect vision. Retinal complications, on the other hand, have the potential to cause a significant effect on the patient's vision. Hydroxychloroquine binds to the pigmented retinal epithelial layer and may lead to permanent visual loss. Initially, retinal changes are asymptomatic, hence the need for screening as described earlier in the article. Further retinal deterioration may lead to a "bull's-eye" lesion, which involves a central patchy area of depigmentation of the macula with a concentric ring of pigmentation around it. The patient may describe letters dropping out of words while reading, photophobia, visual field defects, and flashing lights. Major risk factors for developing retinal complications include daily dosage of the drug, duration of treatment, cumulative dose in excess of 800 g, age older than 70 years, and preexisting liver, renal, or retinal disease. A daily dose of more than 6.0 to 6.5 mg/kg in patients with renal or liver failure is associated with an increased risk of retinal complications.[14]

Sulfasalazine

The most potential serious adverse effect of sulfasalazine is hematologic toxicities. The most common presentation is likely to be leukopenia, affecting between 1% and 3% of patients. Other rare presentations include thrombocytopenia, agranulocytosis, aplastic anemia, and hemolysis in patients with glucose-6-phosphate dehydrogenase deficiency. Even though few data exist on liver toxicity associated with the use of sulfasalazine, some experts recommend estimation of levels of baseline liver transaminases in patients with suspected liver disease.[14]

Methotrexate

Methotrexate is commonly used in the treatment of RA; however, this drug is used in other rheumatologic disorders, which include SLE, psoriatic arthritis, and other rheumatologic disorders. Methotrexate is associated with many serious side effects and toxicities, which require the patients to be closely monitored. Most patients develop adverse events from methotrexate. The most serious of these toxicities are myelosuppression, hepatic fibrosis, and cirrhosis. The main risk factor for developing methotrexate-induced hepatotoxicity is the presence of preexisting liver disease. Patients with preexisting liver disease should not be initiated on the drug, and if suspicion of an underlying liver disorder exists, a liver biopsy should be done first. However, routine liver biopsies on all patients are not indicated. The incidence of elevated alanine aminotransferase and aspartate aminotransferase levels in patients receiving methotrexate is 14% and 8%, respectively. These elevations in transaminases resolve within a month of discontinuing the drug. Risk factors for the development of methotrexate-induced myelosuppression include folic acid deficiency and renal insufficiency. Care must be taken when antifolate agents, such as trimethoprim, are used. Folic acid supplementation is therefore recommended for all patients taking methotrexate. A baseline CBC and determination of levels of creatinine, liver transaminases, and albumin are also recommended on all patients before initiation of therapy and should be repeated every 4 to 8 weeks.[9] Taking a thorough history of alcohol consumption is of great importance in screening for patients with underlying liver disease, and may also be used as an opportunity to counsel these individuals on strict avoidance of alcohol.

Methotrexate-induced pneumonitis is also a serious complication, which occurs in 2% to 8% of patients.[15] This condition is mainly monitored through patient education about symptoms of the disease, which include cough, shortness of breath, and dyspnea on exertion. Acute cases may present with fever, chills, and malaise as well. Practitioners should also screen all patients on their follow-up visits for these symptoms. Pneumonitis may occur at any time during therapy and is linked to some known risk factors, which include age more than 60 years, rheumatoid pulmonary involvement, previous use of DMARDs, hypoalbuminemia, and diabetes mellitus.[16] Once there is a suspicion of pulmonary involvement, further testing is indicated to confirm the diagnosis. Testing includes imaging, spirometry, bronchoalveolar lavage, and lung biopsies. These tests do not have good sensitivities and specificities, and a combination of tests is often required to make a diagnosis. However, once the diagnosis is made, methotrexate should be discontinued. Clinical improvement ensues within days, followed by radiographic improvement after several weeks.[17] Glucocorticoid therapy may also be indicated if there is histologic evidence of hypersensitivity pneumonitis, especially if symptoms persist after discontinuation of methotrexate.

Gold Compounds

Gold compounds are used in numerous rheumatologic diseases including RA, juvenile RA, ankylosing spondylitis, and psoriatic arthritis. Adverse events are common among patients receiving intramuscular gold injections, occurring with a frequency of 87 per 100 patient-years, which leads to the discontinuation of therapy in 26% of patients within the first 3 years.[18] Common complications include dermatitis, stomatitis, hematuria, and proteinuria. Renal complications (proteinuria and hematuria) are caused by a gold-induced membranous nephropathy. This complication tends to be transient and may resolve spontaneously. Discontinuation of gold therapy is also associated with resolution of the renal complications, usually requiring on average 11 months, but may take 2 to 3 years for complete resolution.[19] No glucocorticoid therapy is usually required, and gold may be restarted after resolution of proteinuria at a 50% lower dose.[20] Hematologic complications are rare but are associated with gold therapy. Most complications are related to bone marrow suppression. Pancytopenia carries an incidence rate of 0.5%; agranulocytosis also has been documented, and can occur with the use of oral and parenteral preparations. Thrombocytopenia occurs at an incidence rate of 1% to 3% and is caused by autoimmune destruction of the platelets. Thrombocytopenia may be life threatening and may present with easy bruising or petechiae.

Gold therapy may also lead to several pulmonary complications, the most common of which is interstitial pneumonitis. Patients present with dyspnea and cough in most cases. Some may present with fevers and a rash. Laboratory findings are nonspecific in these cases, but chest radiographs commonly show diffuse interstitial opacities with a predominance in the mid and upper lung fields. Treatment involves discontinuation of gold therapy and corticosteroids in severe cases.[21]

Other rare adverse effects of gold compounds include enterocolitis and neuropathies. Surveillance for complications in patients on gold preparations entails obtaining a baseline CBC, renal function testing, and a urinalysis to test for proteinuria and preexisting renal disease, which would preclude the use of gold. These investigations are repeated every 2 weeks during the induction phase and every 1 to 3 months thereafter.

Azathioprine

Azathioprine is used in the treatment of RA among other rheumatic disorders such as SLE. Gastrointestinal side effects occur frequently in up to 23% of patients. These side effects occur mainly in the form of nausea, anorexia, and vomiting. Mild elevation of liver transaminases occurs in approximately 5% of cases. A more severe complication with the use of azathioprine is myelosuppression leading to an increased incidence of sepsis, severe anemia, and bleeding. Risk factors for myelosuppression include the use of allopurinol, angiotensin-converting enzyme inhibitors, or the presence of renal insufficiency. Azathioprine may also be associated with an increased incidence of malignancies. These malignancies include non–Hodgkin lymphoma, Kaposi sarcoma, cervical cancer, and cancer of the vulva and perineum.

Cyclosporine and Tacrolimus

Cyclosporine and tacrolimus share a common mode of action by selectively inhibiting transcription of interleukin-2, and are used in numerous autoimmune disorders such as RA and systemic sclerosis. These drugs share similar side effect profiles as well, the most common of which is renal toxicity. In most cases renal toxicity is reversible; however, in some cases the side effect progresses and causes chronic renal failure. Elevation of systemic blood pressure may also occur because of renal vasoconstriction. These cases require an immediate reduction in the dose and the possible use of antihypertensives; calcium channel blockers are the treatment of choice, which may reverse the vasoconstriction.

Neurologic effects are common in patients taking cyclosporine and tacrolimus. Some effects are mild, such as tremors occurring in 40% of patients. Other less common but more severe complications include seizures, visual abnormalities, focal neurologic deficits, encephalopathy, and coma.[22] Studies concerning the use of tacrolimus in patients undergoing renal transplantation revealed a dramatic increase in the incidence of diabetes mellitus, occurring more frequently in African Americans than in Caucasians.[23] Surveillance of patients receiving cyclosporine or tacrolimus should involve a baseline CBC and evaluation of levels of creatinine, blood urea nitrogen, and liver transaminases. These tests should be repeated every 2 weeks for the first 3 months and every 1 to 2 months thereafter, with close attention to blood pressure measurements to screen for blood pressure elevation.

Mycophenolate Mofentil

Mycophenolate mofentil, also classified as a DMARD, is used in numerous rheumatic diseases and acts through its inhibitory effects on lymphocytic proliferation. Gastrointestinal symptoms (including nausea, abdominal pain, and diarrhea) are the most common side effects and may be alleviated through dose adjustment. Bone marrow suppression leading to leukopenia requires regular monitoring through routine CBCs after the first 1 to 2 weeks of therapy, then 6 to 8 weeks thereafter if blood counts are stable.

Other Medications

Cyclophosphamide

CYC is a potent immunosuppressive agent used in numerous connective tissue disorders for short-term as well as long-term therapy. This drug has the potential of inducing significant toxic effects on the human body during and after cessation of therapy. The immunosuppressive effects of CYC may lead to infections with opportunistic pathogens. This risk is further increased if therapy is combined with the administration of other immunosuppressive agents such as glucocorticoids. Infection with *Pneumocystis carinii* is of special concern during therapy. Such a risk is significantly reduced with prophylactic therapy using trimethoprim-sulfamethoxazole (Bactrim DS). Patients with sulfa allergies may take dapsone or atovaquone. CYC is also associated with cystitis and bladder cancer through the effects of its toxic metabolites. The incidence of these effects may be decreased with concomitant administration of mercaptoethane sulfonate (mesna), which exists in both a parenteral and an oral formulation.

Surveillance of patients on CYC consists of frequent monitoring of white blood cell counts through obtaining CBCs every 2 weeks. A total white blood cell count of less than $3500/mm^3$ should result in a decrease of the CYC dose. Renal functions and electrolytes should also be checked every 2 weeks to assist in proper dosing of the drug. Urinalysis for the presence of blood should be obtained monthly while taking CYC and annually after discontinuation. Such testing will assist in screening for drug-induced cystitis, malignant and premalignant changes, as well as the occurrence of glomerulonephritis.

Nonsteroidal anti-inflammatory drugs

Nonsteroidal anti-inflammatory drugs (NSAIDs) are frequently used in patients with rheumatologic disorders and exert their action through inhibition of the enzyme cyclooxygenase (COX), which results in improvements of symptoms and signs of inflammation. However, NSAIDs do not change the course of or modify the disease process. The use of NSAIDs is associated with adverse effects, mainly gastrointestinal complications. These patients have a 3 times higher risk of developing serious gastrointestinal complications.[24] It may be possible to mitigate this risk by cotherapy with proton pump inhibitor, high-dose histamine-2 receptor antagonist, misoprostol (a synthetic prostaglandin E_1 analogue), or COX-2 inhibitors in place of the more traditional nonselective inhibitors such as ibuprofen and naproxen. COX-2 inhibitors are associated with fewer gastric complications when used alone; however, when combined with aspirin, the benefits become insignificant.[25] One study showed that the use of enteric-coated aspirin was not associated with a clinically significant reduction of gastrointestinal bleeding when compared with the use of other regular forms of aspirin.[26] Other important adverse effects of NSAIDs include acute renal failure due to renal vasoconstriction, or acute interstitial nephritis and hepatotoxicity. Surveillance in patients using NSAIDs may include obtaining a baseline CBC, urinalysis, and measuring levels of creatinine and liver transaminases. These tests may be followed with annual CBCs and renal function testing as well as symptomatic monitoring for gastrointestinal complications.

Long-term glucocorticoid therapy
Glucocorticoids have been used in the management of rheumatic disorders and connective tissue diseases, and although glucocorticoids are associated with significant improvements in signs and symptoms, long-term therapy is associated with numerous adverse effects. One of the most common side effects is weight gain. Other serious effects include hypertension, hyperglycemia, hyperlipidemia, osteoporosis, avascular necrosis, cataracts, and infections. Avoiding most of these side effects may be accomplished by a continuous effort to decrease the dose of the glucocorticoids.[27] Evidence to support the monitoring of patients on long-term glucocorticoid therapy has not been clear. However, some recommendations have been put forth by expert panels to assist physicians in their surveillance efforts. Such surveillance, however, has not shown itself to be cost-effective but may play a bigger role for patients with underlying risk factors for developing adverse effects.[28]

REFERENCES

1. Lassere MN, Johnson KR, Woodworth TG, et al. Challenges and progress in adverse event ascertainment and reporting in clinical trials. J Rheumatol 2005; 32(10):2030–2.
2. Woodworth T, Furst DE, Alten R, et al. Standardizing assessment and reporting of adverse effects in rheumatology clinical trials II: the Rheumatology Common Toxicity Criteria v.2.0. J Rheumatol 2007;34(6):1401–14.
3. Maradit-Kremers H, Crowson C, Nicola P, et al. Increased unrecognized coronary heart disease and sudden deaths in rheumatoid arthritis. Arthritis Rheum 2005; 52(2):402–11.
4. Fernando MM, Isenberg DA. How to monitor SLE in routine clinical practice. Ann Rheum Dis 2005;64(4):524–7.
5. Naranjo A, Sokka T, Descalzo M, et al. Cardiovascular disease in patients with rheumatoid arthritis: results from the QUEST-RA study. Arthritis Res Ther 2008; 10:R30.
6. Karstila K, Korpela M, Sihvonen S, et al. Prognosis of clinical renal disease and incidence of new renal findings in patients with rheumatoid arthritis: follow-up of a population-based study. Clin Rheumatol 2007;26:2089.
7. Summey B, Yosipovitch G. Prevention of osteoporosis associated with chronic glucocorticoid therapy. Arch Dermatol 2006;142:82–90.
8. Leandro MJ, Isenberg DA. Rheumatic diseases and malignancy—is there an association? Scand J Rheumatol 2001;30(4):185–8.
9. Saag KG, Teng GG, Patkar NM, et al. American College of Rheumatology 2008 recommendations for the use of nonbiologic and biologic disease-modifying antirheumatic drugs in rheumatoid arthritis. Arthritis Rheum 2008;59(6):762–84.

10. Konttinen L, Honkanen V, Uotila T, et al. Biological treatment in rheumatic diseases: results from a longitudinal surveillance: adverse events. Rheumatol Int 2006;26:916–22.

11. Yazici Y, Erkan D, Paget SA. Monitoring by rheumatologists for methotrexate-, etanercept-, infliximab-, and anakinra-associated adverse events. Arthritis Rheum 2003;48:2769–72.

12. Bongartz T, Sutton AJ, Sweeting MJ, et al. Anti-TNF antibody therapy in rheumatoid arthritis and the risk of serious infections and malignancies. JAMA 2006;295:2275.

13. Listing J, Strangfeld A, Kary S, et al. Infections in patients with rheumatoid arthritis treated with biologic agents. Arthritis Rheum 2005;52:3403.

14. American College of Rheumatology Ad Hoc Committee on Clinical Guidelines. Guidelines for monitoring drug therapy in rheumatoid arthritis. Arthritis Rheum 1996;39(5):723–31.

15. Kinder AJ, Hassell AB, Brand J, et al. The treatment of inflammatory arthritis with methotrexate in clinical practice: treatment duration and incidence of adverse drug reactions. Rheumatology (Oxford) 2005;44(1):61–6.

16. Alarcón GS, Kremer JM, Macaluso M, et al. Risk factors for methotrexate-induced lung injury in patients with rheumatoid arthritis. A multicenter, case-control study. Methotrexate-Lung Study Group. Ann Intern Med 1997;127(5):356–64.

17. Searles G, McKendry RJ. Methotrexate pneumonitis in rheumatoid arthritis: potential risk factors. Four case reports and a review of the literature. J Rheumatol 1987;14(6):1164–71.

18. Van Jaarsveld CH, Jahangier ZN, Jacobs JW, et al. Toxicity of anti-rheumatic drugs in a randomized clinical trial of early rheumatoid arthritis. Rheumatology (Oxford) 2000;39(12):1374–82.

19. Hall CL, Fothergill NJ, Blackwell MM, et al. The natural course of gold nephropathy: long term study of 21 patients. Br Med J (Clin Res Ed) 1987;295(6601):745–8.

20. Klinkhoff AV, Teufel A. Reinstitution of gold after gold induced proteinuria. J Rheumatol 1997;24(7):1277–9.

21. Tomioka R, King TE Jr. Gold-induced pulmonary disease: clinical features, outcome, and differentiation from rheumatoid lung disease. Am J Respir Crit Care Med 1997;155(3):1011–20.

22. Gijtenbeek JMM, van den Bent MJ, Vecht Ch J. Cyclosporine neurotoxicity: a review. J Neurol 1999;246:339–46.

23. Neylan JF. Racial differences in renal transplantation after immunosuppression with tacrolimus versus cyclosporine. FK506 Kidney Transplant Study Group. Transplantation 1998;65(4):515–23.

24. Gabriel SE, Jaakkimainen L, Bombardier C. Risk for serious gastrointestinal complications related to use of nonsteroidal anti-inflammatory drugs. A meta-analysis. Ann Intern Med 1991;115(10):787–96.

25. Lanza FL, Chan FK, Quigley EM, et al. Guidelines for prevention of NSAID-related ulcer complications. Am J Gastroenterol 2009;104(3):728–38.

26. Kelly JP, Kaufman DW, Jurgelon JM, et al. Risk of aspirin-associated major upper-gastrointestinal bleeding with enteric-coated or buffered product. Lancet 1996;348(9039):1413–6.

27. McDonough AK, Curtis JR, Saag KG. The epidemiology of glucocorticoid-associated adverse events. Curr Opin Rheumatol 2008;20(2):131–7.

28. Da Silva JA, Jacobs JW, Kirwan JR, et al. Safety of low dose glucocorticoid treatment in rheumatoid arthritis: published evidence and prospective trial data. Ann Rheum Dis 2006;65(3):285–93.

Index

Note: Page numbers of article titles are in **boldface** type.

Prim Care Clin Office Pract 37 (2010) 805–815
doi:10.1016/S0095-4543(10)00087-4
0095-4543/10/$ – see front matter © 2010 Elsevier Inc. All rights reserved.

primarycare.theclinics.com

United States Postal Service

Statement of Ownership, Management, and Circulation
(All Periodicals Publications Except Requestor Publications)

1. Publication Title	2. Publication Number	3. Filing Date
Primary Care: Clinics in Office Practice	0 4 4 - 6 9 0	9/15/10

4. Issue Frequency	5. Number of Issues Published Annually	6. Annual Subscription Price
Mar, Jun, Sep, Dec	4	$190.00

7. Complete Mailing Address of Known Office of Publication (Not printer) (Street, city, county, state, and ZIP+4®)

Elsevier Inc.
360 Park Avenue South
New York, NY 10010-1710

Contact Person

Stephen Bushing

Telephone (Include area code)

215-239-3688

8. Complete Mailing Address of Headquarters or General Business Office of Publisher (Not printer)

Elsevier Inc., 360 Park Avenue South, New York, NY 10010-1710

9. Full Names and Complete Mailing Addresses of Publisher, Editor, and Managing Editor (Do not leave blank)

Publisher (Name and complete mailing address)

Kim Murphy, Elsevier, Inc., 1600 John F. Kennedy Blvd. Suite 1800, Philadelphia, PA 19103-2899

Editor (Name and complete mailing address)

Barbara Cohen-Kligerman, Elsevier, Inc., 1600 John F. Kennedy Blvd. Suite 1800, Philadelphia, PA 19103-2899

Managing Editor (Name and complete mailing address)

Catherine Bewick, Elsevier, Inc., 1600 John F. Kennedy Blvd. Suite 1800, Philadelphia, PA 19103-2899

10. Owner (Do not leave blank. If the publication is owned by a corporation, give the name and address of the corporation immediately followed by the names and addresses of all stockholders owning or holding 1 percent or more of the total amount of stock. If not owned by a corporation, give the names and addresses of the individual owners. If owned by a partnership or other unincorporated firm, give its name and address as well as those of each individual owner. If the publication is published by a nonprofit organization, give its name and address.)

Full Name	Complete Mailing Address
Wholly owned subsidiary of	4520 East-West Highway
Reed/Elsevier, US holdings	Bethesda, MD 20814

11. Known Bondholders, Mortgagees, and Other Security Holders Owning or Holding 1 Percent or More of Total Amount of Bonds, Mortgages, or Other Securities. If none, check box ▶ ☐ None

Full Name	Complete Mailing Address
N/A	

12. Tax Status (For completion by nonprofit organizations authorized to mail at nonprofit rates) (Check one)
The purpose, function, and nonprofit status of this organization and the exempt status for federal income tax purposes:
☐ Has Not Changed During Preceding 12 Months
☐ Has Changed During Preceding 12 Months (Publisher must submit explanation of change with this statement)

PS Form 3526, September 2007 (Page 1 of 3 (Instructions Page 3)) PSN 7530-01-000-9931 PRIVACY NOTICE: See our Privacy policy in www.usps.com

---

13. Publication Title	14. Issue Date for Circulation Data Below
Primary Care: Clinics in Office Practice	September 2010

15. Extent and Nature of Circulation		Average No. Copies Each Issue During Preceding 12 Months	No. Copies of Single Issue Published Nearest to Filing Date
a. Total Number of Copies (Net press run)		734	700
b. Paid Circulation (By Mail and Outside the Mail)	(1) Mailed Outside-County Paid Subscriptions Stated on PS Form 3541. (Include paid distribution above nominal rate, advertiser's proof copies, and exchange copies)	329	312
	(2) Mailed In-County Paid Subscriptions Stated on PS Form 3541 (Include paid distribution above nominal rate, advertiser's proof copies, and exchange copies)		
	(3) Paid Distribution Outside the Mails Including Sales Through Dealers and Carriers, Street Vendors, Counter Sales, and Other Paid Distribution Outside USPS®	152	57
	(4) Paid Distribution by Other Classes Mailed Through the USPS (e.g. First-Class Mail®)		
c. Total Paid Distribution (Sum of 15b (1), (2), (3), and (4))	▶	481	369
d. Free or Nominal Rate Distribution (By Mail and Outside the Mail)	(1) Free or Nominal Rate Outside-County Copies Included on PS Form 3541	87	69
	(2) Free or Nominal Rate In-County Copies Included on PS Form 3541		
	(3) Free or Nominal Rate Copies Mailed at Other Classes Through the USPS (e.g. First-Class Mail)		
	(4) Free or Nominal Rate Distribution Outside the Mail (Carriers or other means)		
e. Total Free or Nominal Rate Distribution (Sum of 15d (1), (2), (3) and (4))	▶	87	69
f. Total Distribution (Sum of 15c and 15e)	▶	568	438
g. Copies not Distributed (See instructions to publishers #4 (page #3))	▶	166	262
h. Total (Sum of 15f and g)	▶	734	700
i. Percent Paid (15c divided by 15f times 100)		84.68%	84.25%

16. Publication of Statement of Ownership

If the publication is a general publication, publication of this statement is required. Will be printed in the December 2010 issue of this publication. ☐ Publication not required

17. Signature and Title of Editor, Publisher, Business Manager, or Owner	Date
Stephen R. Bushing — Stephen R. Bushing – Fulfillment/Inventory Specialist	September 15, 2010

I certify that all information furnished on this form is true and complete. I understand that anyone who furnishes false or misleading information on this form or who omits material or information requested on the form may be subject to criminal sanctions (including fines and imprisonment) and/or civil sanctions (including civil penalties).

PS Form 3526, September 2007 (Page 2 of 3)

Moving?

Make sure your subscription moves with you!

To notify us of your new address, find your **Clinics Account Number** (located on your mailing label above your name), and contact customer service at:

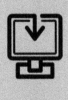

Email: journalscustomerservice-usa@elsevier.com

800-654-2452 (subscribers in the U.S. & Canada)
314-447-8871 (subscribers outside of the U.S. & Canada)

Fax number: 314-447-8029

Elsevier Health Sciences Division
Subscription Customer Service
3251 Riverport Lane
Maryland Heights, MO 63043

*To ensure uninterrupted delivery of your subscription, please notify us at least 4 weeks in advance of move.

Printed and bound by CPI Group (UK) Ltd, Croydon, CR0 4YY

03/10/2024

01040445-0014

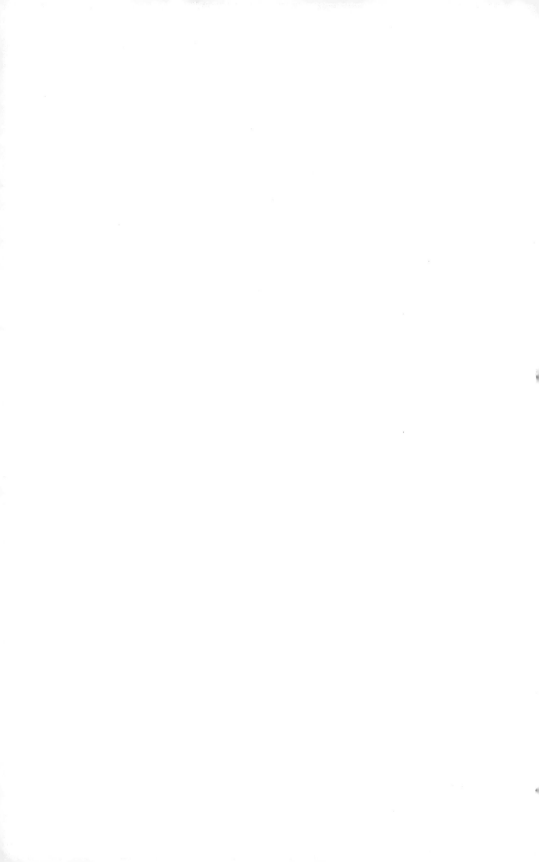